Advance Praise for

The Catching Point Transformation

"Dr. Prologo targets sustainability. He elevates our science-based weight loss programs—by keeping people engaged."

—Arthur Agatston, MD, Author of *The South Beach Diet*

"By leading us past the false promises of weight control by force of will alone, Dr. Prologo provides both empowerment and relief. With experience, expertise, and careful attention to evidence, he converts the frustrating limitations of reliance on will into an actual way paved with genuine understanding."

—David Katz, MD, MPH, Director, Yale University Prevention Research Center-Founder, The True Health Initiative, Author of *How to Eat*

"In this book, Dr. Prologo illuminates the struggles of obese and overweight patients throughthe absolutely fresh lens of aproceduralist, physician, and friend."

—Mark Hyman, MD, 12x *New York Times* Bestselling Author of *Food: What the Heck Should I Eat, The Blood Sugar Solution: 10 Day-Detox Diet,* and many others

"This book is a riveting cheat sheet of new science, new strategies, and new hope for people who are sick and tired of being told they just don't want it badly enough."

—Lesley Paterson, 3x World Champion Triathlete

THE CATCHING POINT TRANSFORMATION

A TWELVE-WEEK WEIGHT LOSS STRATEGY BASED IN REALITY

THE CATCHING POINT TRANSFORMATION

A TWELVE-WEEK WEIGHT LOSS STRATEGY BASED IN REALITY

BY J. DAVID PROLOGO, MD, FSIR, ABOM-D

Post Hill PRESS

A POST HILL PRESS BOOK
ISBN: 978-1-64293-922-4
ISBN (eBook): 978-1-64293-923-1

The Catching Point Transformation:
A Twelve-Week Weight Loss Strategy Based in Reality

Interior graphics by Tiffani Shea

This book contains advice and information relating to health care. It should be used to supplement rather than replace the advice of your doctor or another trained health professional. You are advised to consult your health professional with regard to matters related to your health, and in particular regarding matters that may require diagnosis or medical attention. All efforts have been made to assure the accuracy of the information in this book as of the date of publication. The publisher and the author disclaim liability for any medical outcomes that may occur as a result of applying the methods suggested in this book.

Post Hill Press
New York • Nashville
posthillpress.com

Published in the United States of America
1 2 3 4 5 6 7 8 9 10

This book is dedicated to my beloved mom,
who always encouraged me to read. And to talk good.

Impossible is nothing.

— Muhammad Ali

CONTENTS

PART 2:
Building Your Program

PART 3:
Beyond Fitness

FOREWORD

We are practicing medicine that is a century out of date.

—Dale Bredesen, MD, author of *The End of Alzheimer's*

ONE OF THE MANY JOYS of this profession is the opportunity to guide and mentor others. Dr. Prologo approached me several years ago because his research was leading him to the same conclusions twenty years of functional medicine have led us—that *changes to the body result in changes to the brain.* It has been my pleasure to review Dr. Prologo's work and to discuss his novel approach to age-old problems.

I have treated thousands of patients with interventions based in this thinking—modified depression, anxiety, bipolar disease, psychosis, ADHD, dementia, and more—by changing input to the body from the outside in, primarily through nutrition. Dr. Prologo has likewise treated patients with previously unmanageable conditions, such as phantom limb pain in amputees, by changing the input from the body in order to heal the brain. He has taken this same reasoning to his procedural and behavioral management of obesity, which has resulted in an absolutely fresh, novel paradigm.

In his debut nonfiction work, Dr. Prologo brings a unique combination of training, experience, and expertise to weight loss. He upends traditional thinking by debunking traditional inspirational poster language. "Mind over matter," "change begins on the inside," and "no pain, no gain" are sentiments from the past, according to Dr. Prologo—and I couldn't agree more.

The brain learns, heals, and evolves in response to the body. Signals from our gut, nerves, muscles, and inflammatory system provide a map for our brains. Our brains are wired for survival and will react predictably to external stimuli. In today's world, though—filled with processed foods, multidimensional stressors, and lack of sleep—our brains find themselves backpedaling and fumbling. Trying to survive amongst all of these unnatural stimuli has led to disorders such as obesity, depression, and more.

The Catching Point Transformation presents a new evidence-based approach to weight loss that is founded in changes to the body from the outside in. Dr. Prologo calls for the end of fat-shaming, which is founded in nonsensical claims that patients who are overweight or obese should be able to cure themselves with their minds. Weight loss follows intentional exercise, emotional recovery, and nutrition. Brain function is altered by these interventions, which makes sustainability easier and creates a kinetic success.

Dr. Prologo logically and plainly explains what we in functional medicine know to be true—that our systems break down centrally because of outside influencers. Likewise, we can be repaired, and obesity managed, by modifying those influencers for a retrograde repair of our minds. I am sure that this book will change lives, and I am thankful to Dr. Prologo for allowing me to share in this revolutionary approach.

—Mark Hyman, MD

PREFACE

I ASKED MY MOM one day during one of our many conversations about losing weight, "If you had a gun to your head and your life depended on it—could you stay on this diet?"

"No. No I couldn't," she answered despondently. And then went on to ask if I thought maybe she had a thyroid issue, or her metabolism was slow, or if I could think of any other explanation in the universe that might explain why she couldn't get this done. She was tortured by the idea that she had ostensibly been given the key to weight loss, but that she uniquely couldn't figure out how to turn that key and get the promised results. My mom thought it was her fault. A personal problem with her body, her willpower, or her resolve.

The world outside our home doubled down on my mom's self-blame. The fitness industry was (and still is) run by already-fit-folks. People who have always been lean and have an unlimited number of their programs to sell. They preach from mountains that if all the miserable fat souls *would just do what they do,* they also could be lean. And if they didn't, well—they must not really want to be lean—and that is their fault.

Wait, what?

This is like a group of rich white kids in a private school giving advice to early teens living in a remote village of a third-world country about how to succeed in school and life. Then, when the village resident fails to follow the advice of reading one hour a night because they don't have books or electricity—the private school kids point and say, "Well, that's their fault. I told them what I do and it works for me, so they must not really want it," and "we can't help them if they don't want to help themselves."

Obviously, that would be absurd because the conditions are different. Those from under-resourced nations face challenges that upper middle-class students do not. Therefore, the recipe for success at Prince Peter's School for the Rich and Privileged is not going to translate for kids worried about having enough food and shelter to survive the day. It doesn't mean the village kids lack the willpower or tenacity to stick with the program (and it certainly doesn't mean that the Prince Peter kids are somehow superior). It means the conditions are different.

Likewise, those looking to *make a change* from overweight or obese to lean face different conditions than those who are already lean following the same exercise and diet program. Therefore, no lean person should be pointing their finger saying they provided their recipe for success and anyone who can't follow it is weak-willed and lazy. The conditions are different. It is a different thing to make a change from overweight to lean versus maintaining a lean physique.

The math doesn't lie, they will say. More calories out than calories in equals weight loss. Really? It's that simple? How many of these experts have actually lost a significant amount of weight themselves? I can tell you what the statistics are using that approach: more than one hundred million people tried that last year, and almost no one succeeded even in the short term, let alone with sustained weight loss.

It's not because the math isn't true. *It's because no one can do it.* There are chemotherapy drugs that kill cancer but for some people can't be tolerated because of nausea, blackouts, and so on. Shall we tell those patients who cannot follow the treatment schedule that they must not really want to be rid of their cancer? I mean, the science doesn't lie—those drugs will kill the cancer. So, if they can't tolerate the treatment program, it's their own fault?

It's a bizarre and cruel arrangement, this idea of shaming and condescending people who cannot tolerate diet and exercise programs for long periods of time without ever having walked in their shoes. Without understanding and accounting for their unique challenges and different conditions, but instead labeling them as weak or stupid or lazy.

I have spent my entire adult life studying this phenomenon, and spent many, many years researching this obstacle of diet attrition (the point where people consistently fail available treatment options). I ended up going to medical school because of it, ultimately obtained sub-specialty certification in Obesity Medicine, and performed numerous first in human procedures around this idea of blocking the body's response to dieting. I conducted thousands of hours of formal research trying to understand how to bypass this challenge.

It turns out that those who are already in shape actually *enjoy* those diets and exercise regimens, while those who seek change generally would rather die (see opening sentence) than go through them. Imagine how easy change would be if it were reversed and the obese and overweight populations enjoyed negative calorie balance, instead of feeling like they've been hit by a train.

It also turns out that there is a way to switch sides. To get to the point where running and Yoga and smoothies and cross-fit are actually fun. Once you get there, the rest is easy—and that is the subject of this book.

One more thing. I already have a good job. Everyone is really nice and smart here. So I didn't write this book to make money or trick anyone into buying anything. I wrote it because there are a million more people like my mom and I want you all to know (1) that we now understand you were right about not being able to sustain dieting (and it has nothing to do with willpower or other such nonsense) and (2) there is a way out.

Thank you for your interest and patience, and for the time you spend reading these pages. I hope you can connect with some of what I have written here.

Wishing you all Peace and Love,

David Prologo

J. David Prologo, MD, FSIR, ABOM-D

PART 1:

The Power of the Catching Point

INTRODUCTION—
Mind Over Matter Is Bulls#$%

If you can learn a simple trick, Scout, you'll get along a lot better with all kinds of folks. You never really understand a person until you consider things from his point of view, until you climb inside of his skin and walk around in it.

— Atticus Finch in *To Kill A Mockingbird* by Harper Lee

PATIENTS WHO ARE OVERWEIGHT or obese have higher levels of the hunger hormone, lower levels of the fullness hormone, altered metabolism, learned neural adaptations, and many other clearly defined difficulties to face that lean folks do not. What's more, these difficulties multiply and become more intense as diets progress, making it nearly impossible to sustain any degree of calorie restriction or new exercise over time. When an overweight patient begins to lose weight through dieting, ghrelin (the hunger hormone) goes up, leptin (the fullness hormone) goes down, metabolism slows down, stress hormones increase, and a predictable cascade of resistance is ignited. This backlash is unique to those looking for change and is not present when lean folks undertake the same prescription of diet and exercise.

This backlash is unique to those looking for change and is not present when lean folks undertake the same prescription of diet and exercise.

The purpose of this book is to document this disconnect and get everyone to the same starting line. Science has defined for us exactly what the obese or overweight person is fighting and how those obstacles are not present in their lean counterparts. Attempting to make a change is not the same as exercising to stay fit, and projecting the idea that it is the same has led to widespread prejudicial behavior, unfounded feelings of depression and worthlessness, fat-shaming, and more.

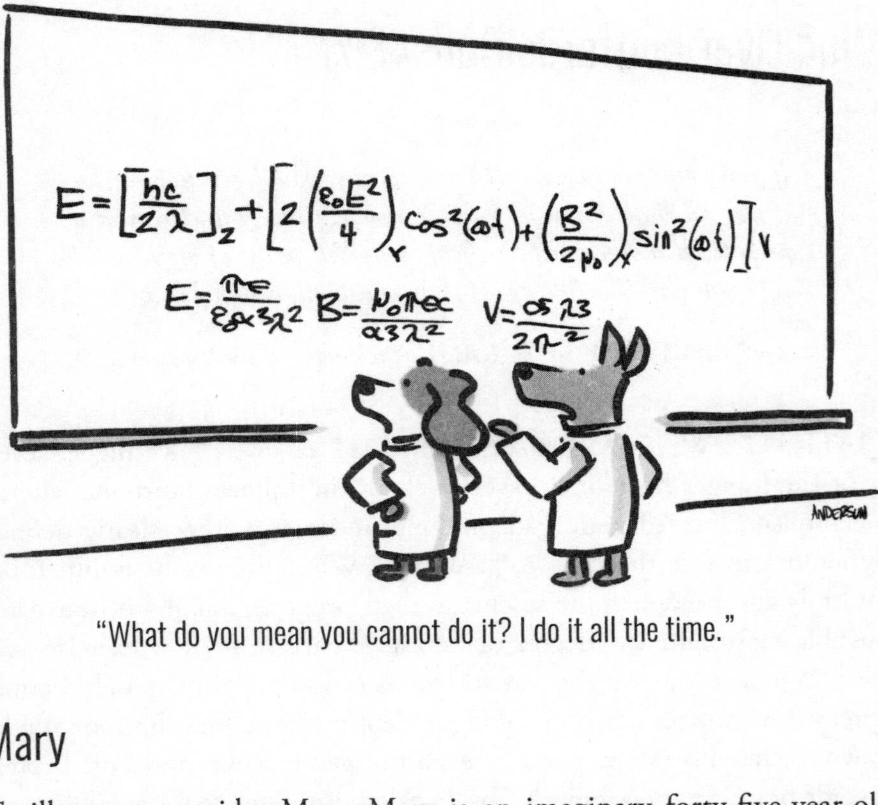

"What do you mean you cannot do it? I do it all the time."

Mary

To illustrate, consider Mary. Mary is an imaginary forty-five-year-old white female whose child is hurt and crying on the other side of a door. The door is unlocked. Mary is of above-average intelligence, and she loves her child. She is terribly upset because she wants to help her child. If I were to put you on the phone with Mary to solve this problem in real time, what would you say?

Most likely, you would say to open the door. Get the child. Case closed. But what if Mary replied that she cannot step toward the door because the floor is unstable and cracking, and each time she moves the crack opens wider, threatening to swallow up her child on the other side. Mary is frozen in place and cannot reach the door. What now?

The point of this scenario is that Mary's challenge is different than the one you pictured in your mind at the beginning. You know what doors look like and how they work in your experience, so you advised her based on that. Open the door. Get the child. When Mary informed you that her conditions were not as simple as you might think, you immediately believed her and started to search your mind for an alternative solution. Good for you.

Imagine if you didn't handle it that way, though. Imagine instead that you did not believe Mary. The floor is not really cracking, you think. The child is not really in danger. Mary must be too lazy or stupid to reach for the door and help her injured child, so she made up this nonsense about the cracking floor. (How ridiculous, though, right? To snap-judge Mary without even knowing her? Stay with me....)

What's more, as you go on in our imaginary scenario, you yourself open doors every day and there is no cracking floor. You have been opening doors your entire life, multiple times a day, and you have never encountered a cracking floor. Obviously, Mary is lying for some reason—probably because she does not really want to get her child. We know she appears upset about the child and is testifying to us with great emotion that she cares about the child, but if that were true, why wouldn't she just open the damn door?

So, you get back on the phone with Mary. You encourage her to open the door so she can care for her child. Exasperated, Mary explains again that the floor is unstable and cracking and when she tries to step it gets worse. She cannot reach the door no matter how bad she wishes she could. You fire back that you have opened doors for years. You are a veritable expert on door opening. All she has to do, you insist, is step forward, grab the handle, and turn. You—the door-opening, imaginary crisis-managing child savior expert—know exactly what it feels like to open a door. Mary should trust you.

As the situation progresses, it becomes clear that you are going to have to do more to convince Mary. Do more to get her across the threshold of this door and to her injured child. Since deep down you are an OK person, and you'd really like to see Mary get through that door, you decide to make videos of yourself walking to doors and opening them. You do it again and again and send them to Mary's phone. "See that!" you say. "See how easy it is!" Mary responds that your instructional videos are great but emphasizes again that her conditions are *different* because of the cracking floor. You roll your eyes. Again with this floor story. (Why is it that we don't believe Mary? Because it never happened to us? Is it impossible that her conditions are different than our own experience? Read on, dear friend. Read on....)

Mary responds that your instructional videos are great but emphasizes again that her conditions are *different*...

"I cannot help this lady if she does not want to help herself," you proclaim to your friends, who also have opened multiple doors many times and don't understand why Mary is saying it is so hard. "Obviously, she does not really want to get to that child."

You

Now, let us add a twist. What would you do if *you* were Mary? What would you do if the person on the other end of the phone insisted on sending you a video of them opening a door? If they rolled their eyes at you when you tried to explain your problem with the floor? Thought you were making it up?

In fact, what would you do if you were stuck like Mary forever? Every day, you encounter more videos and commercials with people smiling and opening doors. You call your friends and loved ones for advice, and they, too, gently try to explain how your story about the floor cracking simply isn't true. It's all in your mind. They too have opened doors so they know how you must feel, and they know how to get that door open. Stop saying that the floor is cracking and get your mind right, they tell you.

"Mind over matter!" they say. "You just have to really want it!" So, you look down. Clearly the floor is cracking, right? No one else seems to think so. "Maybe I am imagining it?" you think. "Maybe I am weak? Maybe I am...worthless?"

After all, getting to your child is important to you, so you grit your teeth and take a step toward the door. All of these people cannot be wrong. But the floor cracks, and you fall. The child remains horrifically out of reach. There is no one on the other end of the phone who believes that the floor is cracking, let alone that it caused you to fall. "You are so full of excuses," they say.

Brutus

Think now what would happen if a cement truck showed up. Brutus the cement guy gets out and surveys your situation. He hears the crying child and sees you on the floor after your fall, desperately trying to stabilize the cracking foundation with your willpower.

You exclaim to Brutus, "I cannot open that door because of this unstable floor!" Imagine your joy when Brutus replies, "Obviously you cannot. Your conditions are different than regular people trying to open doors. You have this extra obstacle. How can anyone expect you to get to that door under these conditions?"

Relief washes over you. Finally, someone understands you. You are not crazy. There is something extra going on with your situation that is different from all those happy people in the door-opening videos.

Brutus acknowledges that no matter how many videos you watch or door-opening experts you consult, your situation is different. You have a floor cracking and breaking every time you move. The people in the videos do not have that to deal with.

Brutus fills the crack with cement. He stabilizes the floor. You walk across, open the door, and pick up your child, who quiets in your arms. (It turns out they weren't hurt, they just missed you.)

As you hold your child and smile, your friends and family slowly gather and congratulate you. "You see? You just had to set your mind to it...."

Matter Over Mind

OK. Now let's talk. Obviously, Mary did not rectify her situation by being mentally strong, and obviously I chose that parable to illustrate the realities of weight loss for you.

The primary lesson to be learned here represents the epicenter of this book. No one believed Mary/you about the cracking floor. Because the helpers on the phone in our story were drawing on their own experiences when it came to opening doors, they refused to consider that *Mary's sit-*

uation may be different. Instead, they did what humans so often tend to do—they attributed negative qualities to Mary, such as lying, confabulating, being weak, stupid, lazy, and more. If just once we could have put the alleged helper in with Mary for only ten seconds, he or she would say, "Holy s#$%, the floor is cracking in here!"

And right there, all the judgment would be off Mary. People would focus on fixing the floor. No longer would they say that Mary was weak, lacked determination, or didn't care about her child. Just ten seconds in Mary's body is all they would need to abruptly change the perception of her situation. What would change in those ten seconds would be an understanding that Mary's conditions are different when compared to people opening doors on solid ground and that those conditions cannot be fixed with any amount of "willpower" or "mind over matter" magic.

If only we could switch bodies when it comes to weight loss. If only we could take a lean, fat-shaming male and put him into the body of an overweight female facing these extra challenges. Force him to try and lose weight and make a change. How great it would be to hear him come back and say, "Whoa, I didn't know you felt like that!"

Just as Mary tried so feverishly to make her well-intentioned callers understand that there was an obstacle to her simply opening the door (the cracking floor), so our weight-loss patients have been trying to articulate their obstacles to us. They have been telling us that their conditions are different and that they cannot lose weight on their own. That their experience with exercise and calorie restriction cannot be the same as these other folks who appear to be enjoying themselves. And we as their helpers, what did we do? We rolled our eyes just like the helper in the example. Again with this story about the cracking floor, we said. Until now.

The Cracking Floor

So, what is the nature of this "cracking floor"? What are the mysterious obstacles that stop overweight persons from being successful with weight loss, and why don't lean people have the same problems? Why should anyone believe someone who claims, "I simply cannot lose weight, no matter what I do," or "I could eat the exact same thing as skinny Sally over there and still gain weight"? Isn't it all just a matter of willpower? Glad you asked.

The Basal Metabolic Rate

Changes in energy expenditure or energy intake trigger powerful responses aimed at restoring that energy balance.

— Jeffrey Sicat, MD, FACE

The first thing an overweight person faces when they try to lose weight by decreasing calories is a response from the body that literally blocks and offsets their efforts. It is a *physiological* response that directly opposes the dieter because excess body fat is a survival advantage. It helps us live through a famine and tolerate temporary food shortages. The body cares about surviving, not looking pretty.

When an overweight person begins a "diet," which usually means some degree of decreasing calories, the first thing their body does is slow down the machine.[1, 2] The body perceives this new decrease in available calories (with or without an associated new energy expenditure from exercise) as a starvation event. In order to survive these adverse conditions, the body is wired to conserve energy. What this means is that our basal metabolic rate (i.e., the way your body handles the food you put in it) decreases so that our body will burn fewer calories in a given day. The metabolism of an overweight individual literally goes down with the onset of their new program. If the dieter doesn't respond in a timely fashion by restoring the missing calories, metabolism slows even more as they lose weight because their body proportions change in a way that signals worsening starvation.[1, 3]

The body perceives this new decrease in available calories... as a starvation event.

To illustrate, consider an abrupt decrease in your income. If you were living on $4,000 a month, let's say, and all of the sudden you went to $2,000—overnight (on a Monday)—you would have to make some adjustments to your daily routine. *In order to survive*, you would have to cut the normal amount of money you spend (your basal rate, as it were) so that you have money for vital things like rent and gas. You would not continue to spend $4,000 a month (or even $3,000) if all of a sudden only $2,000 were available to you. You would hunker down and slow your spending to adjust for this lower amount of money so that you could weather the storm. You would not continue spending at the same pace and bleed out $2,000 a month until you got evicted.

The body sees your diet the same way. If only 2,000 calories are available to you all of a sudden, you cannot continue to burn through 3,000 every day like you did before, because you will starve to death. You need to conserve energy by slowing down your daily burn (calories, after all, are units of energy) for vital functions so you can survive. What happens, then, when the dieter suffers through a calorie-restriction day of salads and water is that the body slows down its burn to offset what you think you accomplished! You think you created a deficit of 1,000 calories, but your body slowed down in response and conserved an extra 500 on the back end, blunting your efforts.

This translates to many of the things we hear our patients say. "My body will not let me lose weight," for example. Or, "I think it's my thyroid," or genetics, or stress, and so on. The patient knows that something happens in their body that fights them when they start this diet, and they try to put it into words for us. "What is the point?" they exclaim. "I cut my calories for days on end and don't lose a pound."

Ahhhh, that makes sense, actually. You suffered in vain because your body fights back and slows its daily burn, and the more you restrict, the more it slows down. The system is fixed against you. The house always wins. Sorry.

There are established equations and more details around exactly how this transpires that are a bit complex for this book. Suffice it to say for now that your basal metabolic rate is the first thing that rises up to block you when you try to make a change in your body weight.

The Hunger Hormone Axis

Research has shown that during dieting, hunger hormone levels increase, making us feel hungry. Even if weight loss is achieved through a diet, the levels stay elevated, and we still feel hungry even after eating.

— Sunil Bhoyrul, MD, Chief of Bariatric Surgery at Scripps Memorial Hospital

The second, simultaneous roadblock the body erects when we excitedly "start our diet" stems from an extensive network of hormones and nerve networks that exist to promote food-seeking behaviors.[4–6] Remember, the body is wired to survive, and to survive we need food. This network is redundant, extensive, and serves as one of the primary reasons why our species still exists. It cannot be overcome with willpower.[1]

Importantly, this system is out of balance in overweight individuals. That means it rebounds and overwhelms any person who sets it off when they decrease calories or start exercise abruptly for purposes of losing weight. To be clear, this system is amplified in persons with excess body weight, resulting in a formidable backlash upon the onset of a new diet—an experience unique to those trying to make a change.

> Dieting increases ghrelin levels. Weight loss increases ghrelin levels.

For example, ghrelin is the hunger hormone. It is produced mainly in the stomach and gets to the brain two ways. First, it activates nerves that connect the stomach and the brain, sending signals to the brain that you are hungry. Second, the stomach dumps this little bugger right into the bloodstream and then the blood carries it to the brain, where it transmits the same message: "Eat!" Dieting increases ghrelin levels. Weight loss increases ghrelin levels.[7–9]

Plainly said, embarking on a diet and losing weight results in *increased* levels of the hunger hormone. A patient who starts at 250 pounds,

1 No doubt somebody knows someone somewhere who overcame this system through sheer mental fortitude. Even if that person exists, and they didn't eventually gain the weight back anyway, we are not talking about them. They are an outlier. We are talking about the other 99 percent of the population.

cuts calories, and begins to lose weight (if they can sustain the calorie cutting long enough to overcome the pushback from basal metabolism) is splashed with increasing levels of ghrelin as resistance to this perceived starvation. What's more, even if the person succeeds somehow in losing weight, the hunger hormone levels remain high! The body is trying to return to its base state of excess body fat in the name of survival. So when the patient (or friend, aunt, mother, etc.) tells us that all they can think about is food, we should believe them. Even if we haven't felt that ourselves. Ghrelin is the second measurable response that leaps up to block dieters—and it is formidable.

Leptin is the fullness hormone. It is produced by fat cells and circulates in the bloodstream to tell your brain when you are full.[10, 11] In obese and overweight humans, this system is reset. Over time the body starts to be resistant to leptin, and patients don't feel as full. (It is somewhat similar to antibiotic resistance developed by bacteria that is overexposed to a given medicine.) Thus, overweight and obese patients don't feel as full as a lean person with the same amount of circulating leptin. It's like having the same amount of oxygen as the next person but never feeling like you can get a good breath.

What's more, leptin levels abruptly drop with a new onset of exercise and weight loss.[12, 13] That's right, exercise and weight loss have been shown time and time again to *decrease* leptin (i.e., fullness) levels and *increase* ghrelin (i.e., hunger) levels. So that feeling of ravenous hunger is real. The body drops everything and focuses on eating as a reaction to diet and exercise. It's an automatic survival response—it thinks if it doesn't get your attention, you will stop eating and die. Leptin is another unique component of the blockade that materializes when an overweight person embarks on a weight-loss crusade.

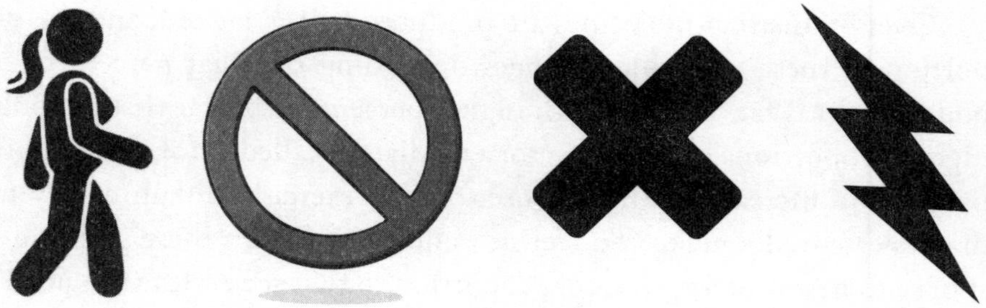

ADIPOSOPATHY (SICK FAT)

The presence of excess fat on the body results in the production of molecules that lead to inflammation, diabetes, arthritis, heart disease, and more.[14] Excess fat on the body also contributes to the resistance felt when diets are begun, in part by participating in the hunger hormone axis as described above, but also by producing a host of inflammatory mediators that make it more difficult to exercise and by affecting the levels of cortisol (the stress hormone) in the blood.

When an obese or overweight person embarks on a new diet and exercise program, they are faced with an uphill battle from day 1. Circulating inflammatory signals produced from excess fat create the need for increased activation energy in order to get started. Said plainly, it is harder to begin and/or maintain exercise because excess body fat responds to it by producing inflammation molecules that make you feel like crap. Real, measurable circulating molecules that the lean person does not have. In fact, it is well known that lean exercisers actually produce hormones that make them feel great—so for them this experience is actually fun!

In addition, obese and overweight patients also have less-active brown fat, which is fat that essentially burns calories "for free" through a process called non-exercise activity thermogenesis (NEAT). Brown fat is a subset of fat tissue found in adult humans, predominantly around our shoulders, upper back, and neck. It has unique features that allow us to burn calories in the background while we go about our normal days, and it can augment attempts to increase energy output in people with normal body composition. In the overweight and obese, this tissue is found in less relative proportion and is often less functional—both effects that are exacerbated by weight-loss attempts. And to add insult to injury, this population loses most of what brown fat function they do have as their initial weight decreases.[15–17]

Over 30 distinct molecules are produced by the fat cell, and the proportion of these molecules changes depending on what percent of our body weight is fat. Patients with higher percentages of fat tissue produce higher proportions of inflammatory mediators called cytokines, and this production increases with the onset of new exercise. Inflammatory mediators essentially make you feel sick and tired. When these go up in response to new exercise—out of proportion to that seen with the same level of exercise in a lean subject—overweight and obese dieters feel a sense of fatigue, malaise (generalized "crappiness"), and even depression that the lean subject does not feel. This response creates a unique challenge that the average trainer or diet coach may not even believe exists. Downstream complications of this response are even more serious and include blood vessel and heart disease, increased risk of cancer, and diabetes.

Again, cortisol is our stress hormone. It is a primitive hormone tied to survival through the "fight or flight" response. Although it certainly has a valuable role in that regard, it also jacks up anxiety when dieters quit. The anxiety overweight and obese people feel as the days go on following the implementation of calorie restriction and new exercise is real, is mediated by cortisol levels that are predictably elevated, and is relieved by food. Moreover, this sequence of events is much more pronounced in patients with higher percentages of body fat. This same process is responsible for "stress eating" and turning to "comfort food" on a lesser scale.

All of these components that originate because the would-be-dieter is starting with excess body fat pile on to make progress that much more difficult compared to a lean person embarking on the same prescription of diet and exercise.

Gut Microbiota

Fat mouse, skinny mouse. Classic experiments in mice show that transplantation of fecal contents (yup, transplants of feces) will make a skinny mouse fat and vice versa.[18, 19] Since then, many of the bacteria in human guts have been shown to exist in—you guessed it—different proportion depending on whether we are fat or skinny.[20, 21]

These different gut flora have different effects on people attempting to lose weight. The obese or overweight person attempting to lose weight faces unique challenges with regard to differential nutrient absorption. Said simply, a banana eaten by an obese individual may translate to 300 absorbed calories, while that same banana in a patient with normal body composition may equal only 150 absorbed calories (that is a bit of an exaggerated difference to make the point that the same food translates to different calories absorbed in different people).

How is that possible? Different gut microbiomes result in (1) increased absorption of carbohydrates, (2) changes in the amount of calories one absorbs from a given food, (3) enzyme changes that result in greater or lesser absorption of a food, and (4) actual physical changes in the gut that "open doors" for calorie absorption. Imagine that bacteria are sitting in the gut as food comes through. Depending on what bacteria are there, the food either gets absorbed (which then has to be either burned or stored as fat) or passes by and exits through the normal route. So when we hear an overweight person report that "I could eat exactly the same food as so-and-so skinny-face and I would gain weight," we should believe them.

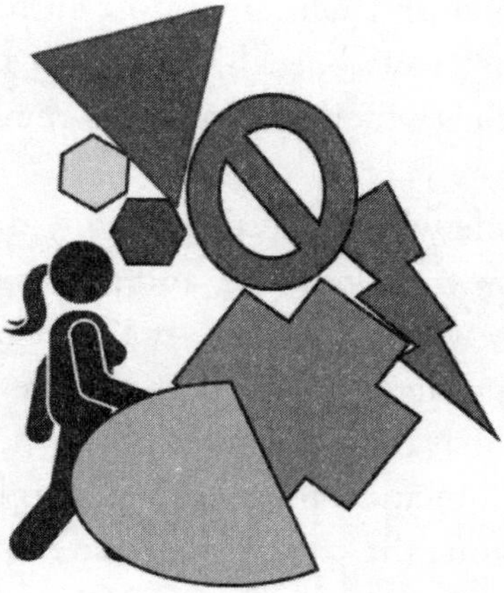

WILLPOWER

Why would anyone think that "willpower" was the culprit in this setting in the first place? Because the lean folks do not feel what the overweight dieter feels when faced with the same stressors. The idea of making a weight change is a completely different project than maintaining one's physique, and overweight and obese folks face absolutely unique, quantifiable entry barriers to healthy living that non-obese patients do not experience.

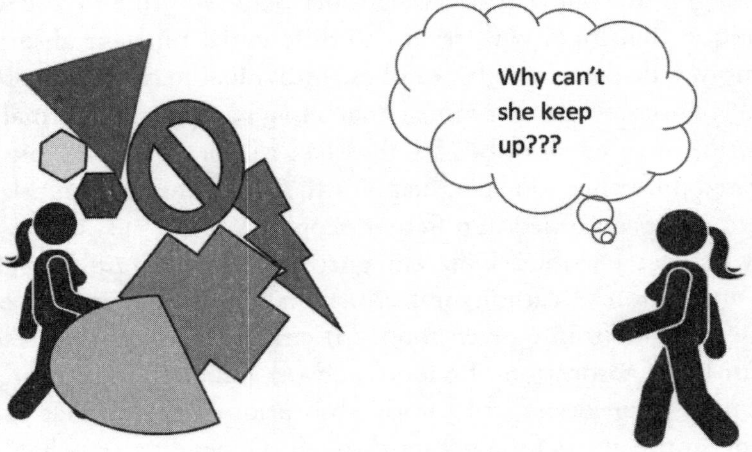

As a result, a powerful misconception was born and exaggerated over time: overweight and obese individuals cannot change their positions in life because of their inability to tough it out through the struggle. Conversely, the lean population (including most authors of mainstream diet and exercise programs) have been blessed with strength, perseverance, and excellence—which is why they can follow these same schedules without quitting. False!

The truth is, no one who succeeds with any diet or exercise program does so through willpower, discipline, and plain old-fashioned grit. That just isn't reality. Those who can follow mainstream programs can do so because they start at a different point than the average overweight or out-of-shape person such that these responses from their bodies are bypassed.

In the absence of a medical intervention, this biological response can only be contained against the current for limited periods of time. It's like holding your breath underwater. We can hold on for a bit, but with time the signals from our brain to seek air, and the changes in our body in response to less oxygen—in the name of survival—cause us to burst to the surface and inhale dramatically. A very similar sequence of events follows the restriction of calories and increased energy expenditure of exercise in the overweight population. The food-seeking response is amplified by a conservation-of-energy response (explained above), which continues to tighten on us until we burst into a fast-food restaurant for relief.

Asking someone to overcome that process with their mind is unreasonable. We don't do it in any other setting. Mind over matter is bull#$%.

CHAPTER 1—

Defining the Catching Point

How, exactly, are we to avoid eating too much? We might eat less than we wish, and [are] hungry all the time, but few of us have the literal or figurative stomachs for that over any length of time. For that very reason, all diets work in the short term, and almost none goes any meaningful distance.

— David Katz, MD, MPH, FACPM, FACP, FACLM

We need to stop thinking about the low Twinkie diet, stop thinking about the number of calories we burn on the treadmill, and start thinking about physiology. …Exercise alters food preferences toward healthy foods…and healthy muscle trains the fat to burn more calories.

— Lee Kaplan, MD, PhD

HOW MANY PEOPLE do you know who have really lost weight? I know of a few: mostly people who have just gotten divorced or dumped, or some of those people on *The Biggest Loser* (and even most of them famously gained it back).[22] But everyday people like us? Not many.

You already know this. You have known for years that you can't lose weight or follow these crazy exercise programs. It's your thyroid. Or genetics. Stress. The devil. It's probably none of those things—but it *is* the way you are built. People who are able to follow most popular, sensationalized exercise and diet regimens are different. They literally, physically, have different hormone profiles and structure that allows them to do it. *But it is a structure that you can have too.*

Expert trainers and fitness gurus also know this. They drone on about "no pain, no gain" and their superhero powers of discipline, dedication, and endurance. They profess how they overcome obstacles that crush the weak and are rewarded with beauty, slim bodies, and nice teeth. The truth, though, is that most available diets work for the beautiful people precisely *because* they are in great shape, not the other way around. They aren't going to work for you in your current state. If you don't believe me, put this book on your shelf and go buy ten of the bestselling, most successful diet and fitness programs, follow them to the letter, and see how you do. Then come back and we'll talk some more.

> No one ever failed a fitness schedule or diet because they ran out of workout options or low-calorie recipes. People succumb to the body's survival signals in the first few days, usually while shopping for rice cakes on the way to fitness boot camp.

Here is the good news. This book will show you how easily you can readjust your body so that you can be successful too. Even better, it's going to be much easier than what you have been doing so far. No more feeling miserable and upset because of your latest impossible food-restriction/exercise plan. We are going to do away with that old-fashioned approach and make the transition refreshing, easy, and fun.

How? What is different about this book? How is this book going to get you to a new point in your life when others have failed? By recognizing that the very drive that motivated you to buy this book in the first place is what will run out first and cause you to quit. Let me explain….

Medical science has shown us that hunger hormones increase during the first few weeks of traditional diet and exercise programs. The onset of the old-fashioned combination of abrupt food restriction and increased exercise is perceived as an assault on the body and flips us into survival mode, resulting in signals from our brain to quit it all. No one ever failed a fitness schedule or diet because they ran out of workout options or low-calorie recipes. People succumb to the body's survival signals in the first few days, usually while shopping for rice cakes on the way to fitness boot camp. This book looks to harness and protect the drive that leads to all these futile "day 1s" by providing the body with what it needs to adjust and evolve in the setting of fitness instead of fleeing the scene to survive. You will nurture your body and train your brain to send new messages back to your body that will condition you to smile and keep on.

We'll get you to a position called the catching point. The catching point is that point in time when the whole thing "catches" and you have that "ah-ha!" moment. You'll shed all the things that make exercise and diet hard, and maybe even make some yoga friends. Sound fun? It's awesome. And it's easy. So bear with me for the short ride through this book, and I promise when you get to the end, you'll be a believer.

Listen, each morning I wake up early before my cases begin. My friend Jon presses snooze four to five times every morning and can barely get to work within 30 minutes of his start time. Jon and I are structured differently. I don't feel like I can't wake up. In fact, I wake up automatically before any alarm goes off because of the way I am wired. I literally have no idea what Jon feels like in the morning because my brain and organs aren't structured like his, *so I don't feel what he feels*. As a result, I may be tempted to say, "I wake up early because God has made me a supreme human being with willpower, determination, and guts to succeed. I choose to work hard and resist the urge to sleep because I am strong." Sure, that would make me feel good, but really—I just wake up.

So the same applies here. No one who succeeds with any diet and exercise program does so through willpower, discipline, and plain old-fashioned grit. That just isn't reality. People succeed because they start at the catching point instead of in no-man's-land, where most of you live (no offense). All you have to do to reverse your futile trend with diet and exercise is get to the catching point *first*.

I know the smiley in-shape people love to tell themselves (and everyone else who will listen) that they have been successful because they possess willpower, strength, focus, and so on and on, but the truth is that they don't resist the urge to eat or be lazy any more than I resist the urge to sleep in. Honestly, are we to believe that these people who go to the gym six times a week, drink smoothies, tan, surf, and smile feel miserable? They do not, because at some point in their lives they got over the hump, and now it's fun. The point of this book, actually, is to show you how to adjust your body so that diet and exercise will be as effortless for you as waking up early is for me.

This is a different goal than you are used to—I should say that up front. Getting to the catching point is an entirely different process than trying to follow someone else's diet and exercise program, and it won't be a pristine, predetermined schedule (more on this in chapter 4). The message here is that in order to become what you hope to be physically, you can't just buy a membership or program and start doing it like "they" do. That is unreasonable. I mean, if I wrote a book entitled *The 12 Steps of Cardiac Bypass*, would you think it reasonable to buy that book and start doing heart bypass surgery? Probably not (I say "probably" because no doubt someone would). The point is, it takes more than a description of the steps involved to effectively perform cardiac surgery—you need some prep work. Likewise, a book detailing a diet and workout schedule is no more effective for weight loss to the untrained person than a description of how to do surgery is for a college freshman.

The majority of "how to be successful" at whatever books are written by people who are already there. This makes some sense because they have knowledge regarding whatever it is they are doing, *but it rarely translates into useful advice for the average human* because there is always something they have and you don't—which is left out of the magic formula. For example, people with $10 million are in a club that you probably don't belong to. If you try to follow the advice in a book called *How to Make $10 Million in One Year*, it is not likely that you will end up with $10 million, because you are starting on the outside. There is no direct route from the average worker to $10 million, except the lottery—and just as the advice in the $10 million book is really a description of steps taken by people who already have money in the bank and an MBA, most fitness schedules are programs followed by people who have been athletes all their lives or who study diet and exercise for a living. In order for you to be successful with any of these fitness programs, you must first "get some money in the bank" and even the playing field. You must get yourself to the catching point.

> The message here is that in order to become what we hope to be physically, we can't just buy a membership or program and start doing it like "they" do. That is unreasonable.

A study was done using 67 independent data sets from 12 countries over two years to try and determine what it was that transformed people to physically active lifestyles.[23] Do you know how many things they found that correlated with physical activity change? Two. That's it: two. And one was the onset of motherhood. The other, which they called "intention," is the subject of this book. It is that rare feeling of *choosing* positive lifestyle elements because you *want* to. Grinding it out against your wishes won't work. Readjusting your likes will.

Imagine any activity in your life that you know well. Your work, your hobbies, your household chores. Now imagine explaining how to do those things to someone that just arrived from the moon who barely speaks your language. In fact, don't even explain it—just give them a schedule of what to do and have them start. I mean, it's the same schedule you follow and you are fine, right? I'm sure they understand the dangers of a hot stove or standing on the plate during a pitch or putting their hands in the trash compactor.

Of course they don't. You would have to provide them with some basic knowledge of what you do, then have them do it for a bit to learn and understand the ins and outs of how you do it successfully. Over time they would start to get it and you would be able to step back. You'd see them gain momentum as they bumped and waded through on their own—learning the subtle things you may have had difficulty putting into words. At some point they would become independent and the task would be *easier* for them, at which point they would likely be able to follow the schedule that seemed so undoable on day 1 without a hitch.

This program focuses on changing *you* in that same way so that when you *do* try to join the next diet trend, you will have the necessary prep work and it will catch. Traditional bestselling shred-your-abs programs are tailored for people who have already reached the catching point, for those who *live* on the other side of the catching point. For them (and for you someday), these programs are easy and enjoyable. In order for you to feel like *that*, unlike the miserable experience of trying to follow these things from where most of us start, you've got to get yourself to the same starting line so that you can share in the momentum and stop swimming upstream.

For the sake of illustration, it bears mentioning at this point that the fitness industry (particularly bodybuilders) knew about low-carb diets for *years* before Dr. Atkins introduced the subject to the general public. This book is similar in that the concept it outlines is well known to the experts, but it undercuts the need for miracle weight-loss products every six months. (Let's face it—the money is in the treatment, not the cure.) Personally, I have been blessed with a day job that I love, so I am not interested in being a weight-loss mogul. I wrote this book because I have watched too many of my friends and relatives spiral down in this trap over the years, and I want them and you to know there is a way out.

The concept of the catching point is illustrated in the figures below. In figure 1, "A" marks the catching point and "B" marks the place most of us dream about. "B" is the place we hope to reach when we follow wellness books and programs and fad diets that feature these people on the cover. *"A" is where successful people start.* The people who write these programs and the athletes who can follow them have a huge head start compared to normal, everyday people and as a result have a totally different experience when they embark on day 1. For them the first week is fun and easy, and they don't feel hungry. They feel refreshed, energized, and healthy, as opposed to hungry, tired, and crabby—because they are coasting downhill from the first day!

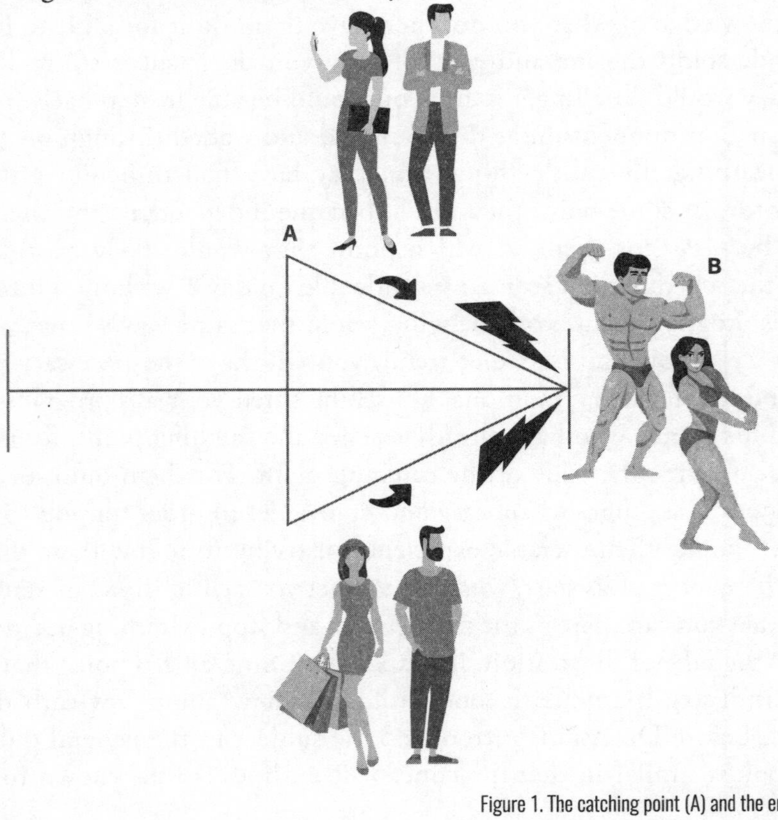

Figure 1. The catching point (A) and the end point (B).

Most of us, on the other hand—in fact 80 percent of Americans—live to the left of the catching point, as shown in figure 2.[24] We gaze with envy at the people for whom all of this is so easy. In fact, *we gaze right past the catching point* and never see it. We don't even know it's there because the allure of being beautiful, in shape, and feeling good is so dizzying and because 99 percent of what is written regarding fitness refers to the glorious trip from A to B.

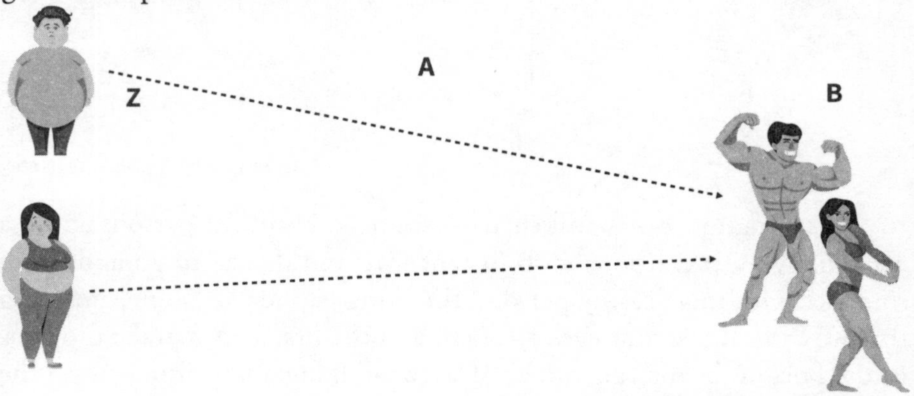

Figure 2. The point of view for the rest of us.

Sadly, we head off toward what looks like a lot of fun. I mean, who doesn't want to be fit and happy and healthy? Because of the path we choose to get there, though, we keep failing, quitting, and bouncing back to square one—as shown in figure 3.

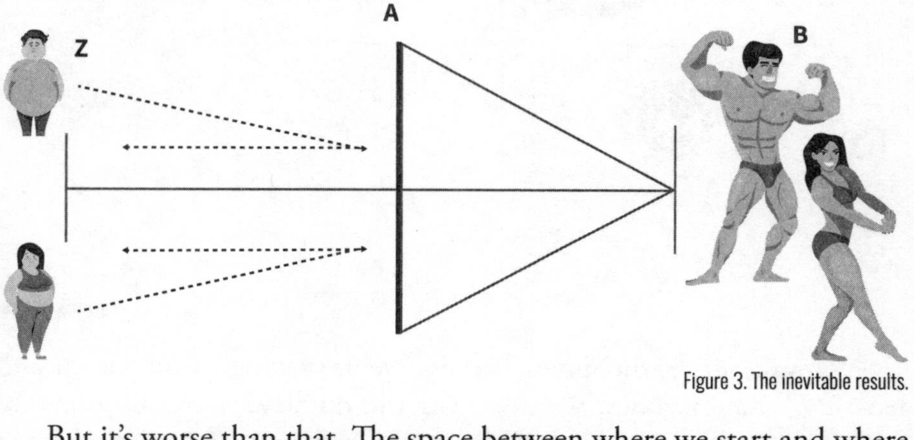

Figure 3. The inevitable results.

But it's worse than that. The space between where we start and where they start ("they" being those obviously in-shape people for whom all of this is easy) is treacherous, as seen in figure 4.

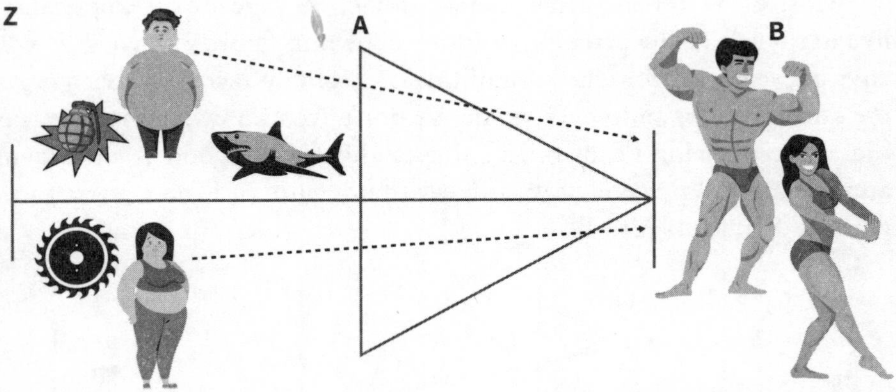

Figure 4. The treacherous space between.

This situation can be likened to seeing a beautiful person across a canyon. We feel delirious with instant love and decide to go and make romance with this dreamy person. The thing is, they are so mesmerizing that we cannot take our eyes off them and the first step we take drops us to the bottom of the canyon, or, if we are talking about fitness, into the treacherous space between us and the catching point, as in figure 5.

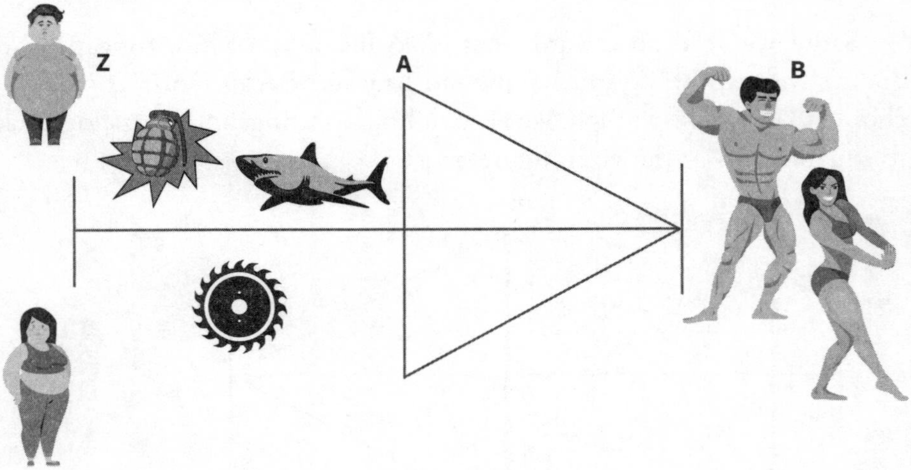

Figure 5. Failure!

We wake up at this point because we are falling to our death and have unpleasant feelings. We give up on this dumb idea to make romance with the dreamsicle (or lose weight, or get in shape), and we climb back to where we started. I mean, after all we obviously can never accomplish anything like this because of our genetics, or thyroid, or whatever.

The thing is, though, after a few months we catch sight of our love muffin again—and guess what? We become mesmerized, decide we have to be with them, step off the cliff, wake up, climb back to the starting point....

And so it goes for many, many people in the pursuit of fitness for the rest of their lives. You can't go directly from Z to B. It cannot be done. You will get eaten by a shark.

What you can do, though, in order to break this cycle of "starting your diet," failing, starting again, and so on is read the instructions in this book *and get yourself to that point A.* Once at the catching point, the great and mysterious secrets that all these other people seem to know will be revealed to you as well. The words and pictures in fitness programs will become understandable to you, and you—after all those failed attempts—will join the army of beautiful people for whom fitness and diet are easy and fun.

You can't go directly from Z to B. It cannot be done. You will get eaten by a shark.

The goal of this book is to get to that point where fitness trends (hot yoga, kickboxing, CrossFit, etc.) will apply to you. In order to do that, you've got to focus on the stepping-stones to the other side of the figurative canyon *first* (figure 6); then you can look up when you are in reach of your long-term goals, or loves. If you take your focus off the stepping-stones—focus off the catching point at A—and try to go directly to the other side, you will likely stumble and end up back at the beginning. So *do* focus on getting to the catching point *only*, regardless of what you think you see at B.

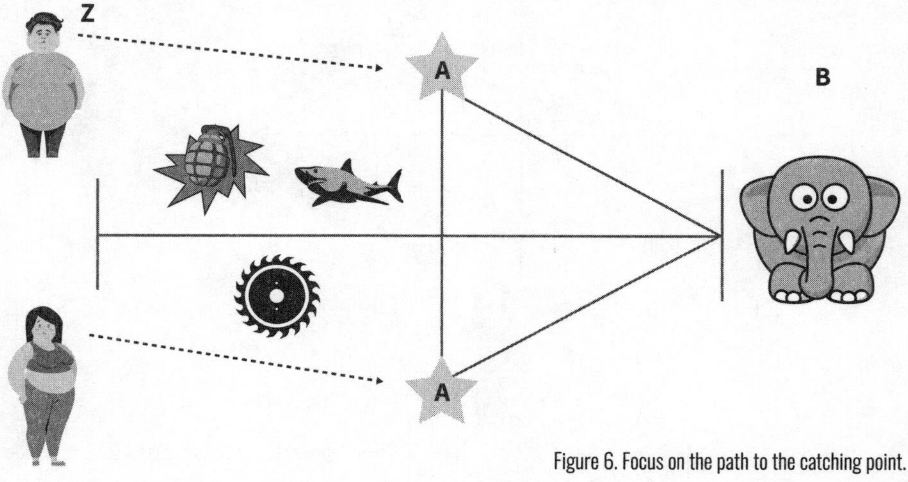

Figure 6. Focus on the path to the catching point.

It is important to point out here that fitness trends change for the same reasons that hairstyles come in and out; skinny jeans are fashionable, then not, then fashionable again; and so forth—because it's fun! These trends emerge because the people who live beyond the catching point get bored with the same old routines (or the same clothes or hairstyles), and it is fun to do something different. They are not invented with the intention of transporting people from Z to B. They emerge to entertain the A-to-B people, just like Pandora bracelets or Birkenstocks (if you are under 45, just stick with the bracelet comparison). But darn heck if we won't buy into the latest trend and see if for some magical reason, this new exercise will catapult us right to B.

No more. After following the instructions laid out in this book, you will be at a new point in your life. You will be trained to understand the fitness world, to participate in it, to enjoy it, to actually do it and get real results. This trip will not be unpleasant. It is not accomplished with the "no pain, no gain" mentality (that, again, is for A-to-B people and is misleading anyway—more on that later). This program will take advantage of changes in your body following exercise so that you feel refreshed, energetic, and motivated. The workouts will get you to the catching point. Once there, you can dust off your diet books and revolutionary exercise programs and blow through them with ease. You can coast, as shown in figure 7.

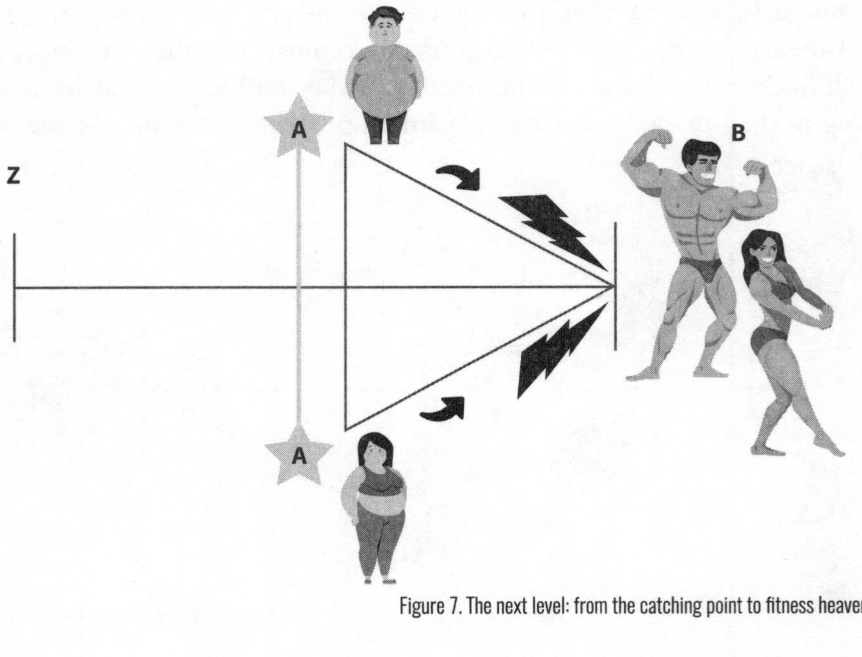

Figure 7. The next level: from the catching point to fitness heaven.

CHAPTER 2—

What You've Been Missing

> *I have come to appreciate that designing and implementing rest and types of rest is perhaps more important than work and the types of work.*
>
> — Dan Pfaff, Olympic track and field coach

WHEN YOU EXERCISE, it's like swallowing a stick of dynamite. Wastes build up, muscles are weakened, your nervous system is shocked, you get dehydrated, and stress hormones are produced.[25–32] The traditional teaching, then, is to push through this feeling and swallow some more dynamite on day 2. And 3, and 4, and so on (until you quit).

In the twenty-first century, though, science has shown us that this bullheaded approach is neither necessary nor effective. The road to success is paved with changes harnessed through *peaceful, individual recovery from exercise.* So what you have been missing is (1) an individualized strategy for knowing when to rest and when to work out so that you can stay on a program for more than a week, and (2) a focus on and understanding of rest and recovery.

Individualized Strategies

People are different.

Consider your children, if you have children. If you don't, please indulge us here, or perhaps reflect on your own childhood. Generally speaking, parents want their children to be happy—to be well adjusted, have rewarding careers, loving spouses, and so on. At the same time, most parents will attest that the road to this happiness for their children is a moving target. The "program" that we have our kids on which we hope will lead to their happiness is constantly changing as our children's personality traits and interests emerge. Oh, and if you have more than one child you will almost certainly notice that your approach becomes individualized to each one. We have some principles that we want to pass on to them (go to college, go to church, be kind), but largely we are reactive based on how they carve out their individual lives. One will be temperamental, one will be free-spirited, one will be neat, one messy, and so forth. The idea, then, is to instill some global principles that will allow them to make good decisions in their own lives without trying to follow a script to the letter. I cannot, for example, treat my son with the same intensity my daughter so easily absorbs. So we try to be flexible in order to get them to the same end point (happy adult lives) through different paths, because they are different from one another. *People are different.*

Likewise, the path to the catching point will be different for each of you, and just as a book outlining 18 years of rigid daily instructions couldn't reasonably be applied to every child in a normal society, so programs for diet and weight loss cannot be blindly, generally applied to people with any hope for success. The catching point program has built-in changeability so that you can determine your course to the end point as your life changes, your motivation waxes and wanes, your body rebels, your mind changes, and so on. But just as you stick to a few important principles when raising your children despite their different personalities, so shall we stick to a key principle in the catching point program: rest. You'll have the flexibility you need to be successful, but we won't waver on this one vital principle, because you can't do it without it.

Another way to illustrate the point that each person must be treated just a bit differently in order to get a group of people to the same goal (in our case the goal of resting enough to change our bodies and make progress with our diet and exercise) is rooted in the basic principles of management. When my son was nine, I coached his basketball team—and I sucked at it, but I learned this principle in the end. (Unfortunately for my son, we went 1–15 while I was processing this point.)

Each practice I would show up with a clipboard and rigid plan for this group of nine-year-old boys. I'd hold them all to the same standards of dribbling, shooting, running, and so forth and run them all through the same drills, rigidly. I applied this practice program and coaching philosophy to all 10 of them in the same exact way over 12 weeks, and here is what happened. One kid of the 10 excelled *because his skill set was already there*. The remaining 9 tried like the dickens to fit their skill sets into my rigid program for which they were not prepared, all the while becoming progressively frustrated and disgruntled and discouraged. One of the dads, Tom, quietly tried to make this point to me. He said, "You've got to get them *all* there, each along their individual paths, using each one's unique strengths." At that time, though, I preferred to try and apply the same blanket program to all the boys, then say that the faltering ones were lazy or dumb or just not cut out for basketball. (By the way, many of those boys went on to become great basketball players.)

So how will you do what Tom suggested? You will learn to hear your individual body's feedback and react appropriately. NASCAR drivers do this, as an example. They recognize the need for pit stops. They know they can't drive a 500-mile race on the same tires because the tires wear down, so they stop periodically during the race and change them, but not according to some preset schedule. They stop according to how the car is performing, how the race is going, and according to the gut instinct of the driver—as will you when you collect your rest and change according to how your body feels and your schedule changes.

You've missed this so far because most diet and fitness books are basically rearranged collections of the same generic instructions. They describe a weight-loss program that may be effective for the people whose skill sets and capacity are already at a certain point—the catching point—and imply that those who are unable to follow the program are lazy or dumb or just not cut out for fitness. The truth, though, is that trying to apply that same program to every individual is bound to fail because each person's recovery will be different. What we aim to do through *this* program is to get each one of you to focus on the in-between changes according to your own personalities, lifestyles, stressors, and motivations, and get everyone to the catching point so that your skill sets will be in place for success in the future.

The Reasons for Focusing on Rest and Recovery

Each time the body undergoes a round of exercise, it will try to adapt, to change for the better, to evolve and be leaner, stronger, and happier. In order to change your body structure, then—to reach the catching point—you must focus on rest, maximizing off days, and banking recovery changes. Accumulating energy and change *in between* workouts will change your body so that you will be able to follow whatever exercise and diet program you want. This will require flexibility over the next 84 days, and it will require rest.[2] You must accumulate these changes and use them as a bridge to the catching point, as shown in figure 8. The rectangle bricks represent the changes you are after. They will protect you from failure, keep you feeling strong, and give you safe passage to the catching point.

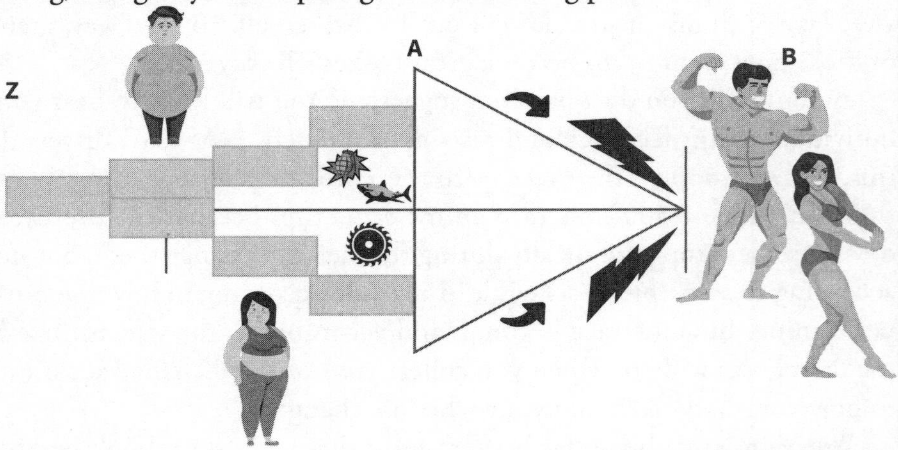

Figure 8. The bridge to the catching point.

Specific things happen during exercise and exercise recovery. So well-known are the changes that occur in between workouts that athletes and fitness folks in the know purposefully capture this process as part of their training.[33] New baselines are established. Red blood cells are replenished, more efficient heart rates and blood pressures are established, stress hormones are decreased, calcium is put into bones, muscles change their structure, metabolic rates are increased, circulating fat and glucose are decreased, immune systems are strengthened, and overall well-being is improved.[34–36]

These changes occur with a real-time feedback loop that lets you know where you are, just like a bar in a video game that tells you how much

2 That's 12 weeks, or 3 months, but it's important to think of this program in individual days. You'll see why as you read further.

life your character has left. That is, in many video games the main character runs around trying to beat levels but slowly runs out of energy, or ammo, or whatever. You have to find something to replenish your supply before you move on. If you just start the game and run your guy forward without paying attention to refuel options, you will pretty quickly die and go back to the beginning. Similarly, most folks mistakenly think that because you miss a workout, eat some cake, or feel like crap, you should bail and start over some other time—when in fact you just need to find a mushroom or a magic coin to charge up. These energy sources are available in life by *delaying and modifying* the next workout and *supplementing* your diet. Likewise, if you ignore your recovery signals and hit the gym before these changes occur, you are sealing your own short-term fate and may end up worse off than when you started.

> The flower needs the water, but more importantly it needs the time in the sun following the water application to restructure itself and bloom.

Imagine a new flower you bring home from the Piggly Wiggly grocery store to brighten up the kitchen. You water it because you want it to bloom, grow, and be beautiful. Then you water it again, and again, and again—without leaving adequate time in between for the flower to absorb the water, take in light, and change. The flower needs the water, *but more importantly it needs the time in the sun following the water application* to restructure itself and bloom. The water itself, like exercise, is there to *induce* change. If you water again before the changes have occurred, the flower will drown and die—and you will quit your exercise program (figure 9).

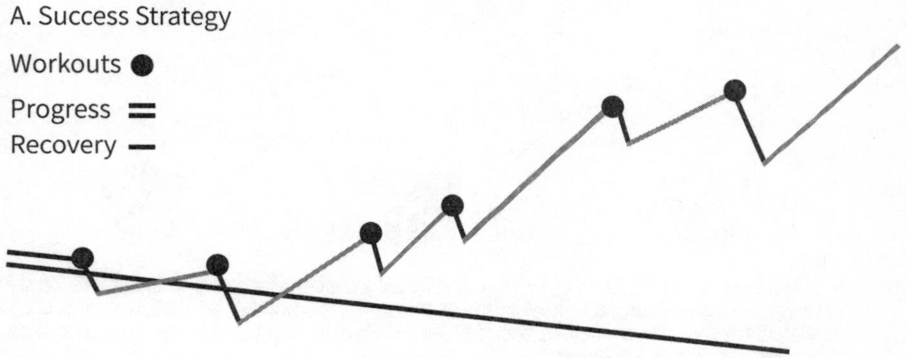

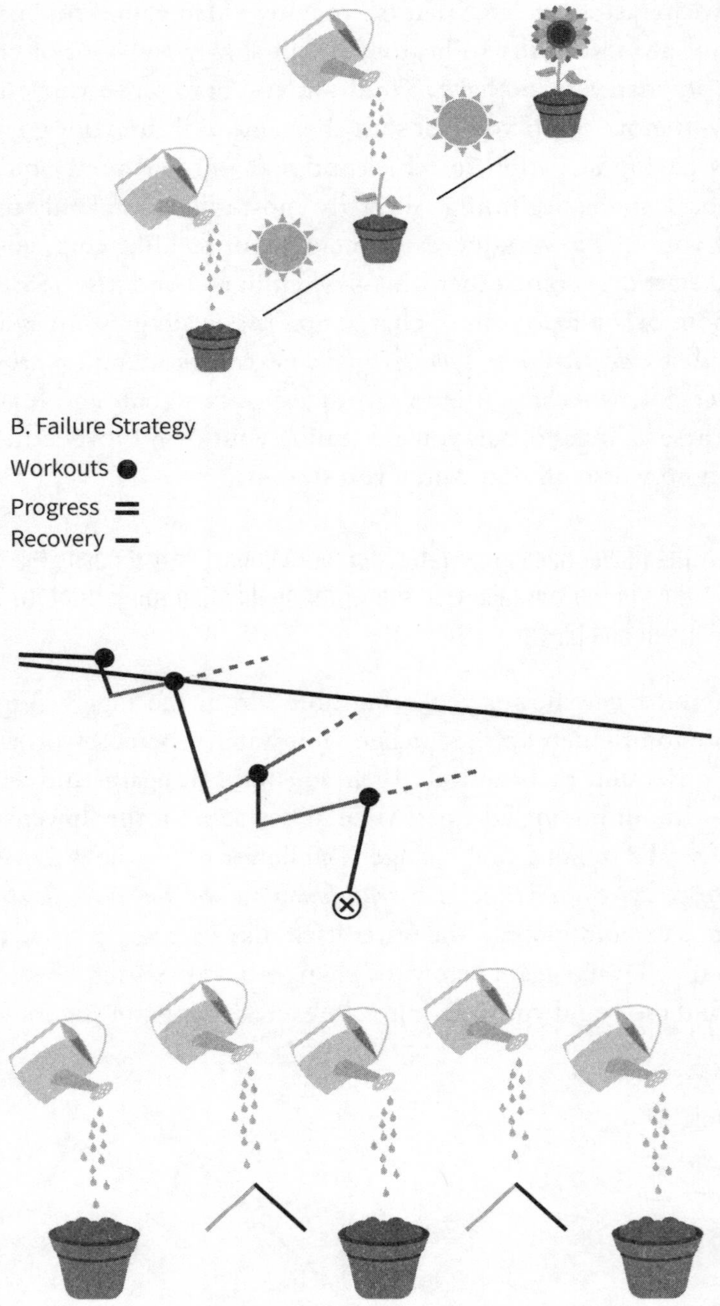

Figure 9. To be successful, it is critical to time your workouts at the end of recovery, allowing time for the application of stress through exercise—or "watering"—to induce change. Traditional programs usually just schedule workouts in a grid, without considering individual recovery time, so the workouts come too soon, before recovery is complete—leading to a downward spiral, or a dead flower.

What is this timeline for recovery, then? It varies, which is what ultimately necessitates a responsive, adjustable, flexible program like the catching point.30, 31 We know that muscles burn calories and synthesize protein for at least 48 hours after your workout, changes occur in your heart and blood vessels for 48 to 72 hours, stress hormones are up for 18 to 24 hours, and inflammatory changes persist for 24 to 72 hours.[37–40] All of these processes give you feelings of soreness, fatigue, motivational drops, or even depression. The key will be for you to recognize this feedback and time your workouts appropriately.

The goal of this program is to harness and nurture these changes through rest, dietary supplements, and conditioning your brain. You need those rectangle boxes from figure 8. Imagine that your task, instead of losing weight, is to dig a 10-by-10-foot hole, and each foot that you dig uncovers a new tool. So you begin digging with your bare hands. After a day or so you get a foot down and find a shovel. Then you continue digging with your shovel and hands for a few more days (or even a week, or two weeks if you are obstinate) until you get bored, your hands hurt, you get a blister, someone invites you to a cookie party, or you pass out from hunger. At this point, *you throw the shovel back in the hole* and go eat some cheeseburgers. Then a few weeks later, you go to a new spot and start all over! What!? Wouldn't it be better if you brought the shovel home with you after lunch at the cheeseburger shack? So you have it when you decide to go back to hole digging?

The mistake you are making is never collecting the tools. Each time you begin again you are back to square one with your bare hands. In the catching point program, your aim will be to collect the tools so when you ultimately begin a traditional exercise program, you have something different with you that will allow you to succeed. By accumulating points during the catching point program (to be explained later), you will accumulate change. You want to have a bunch of rectangular boxes full of tools so that digging the hole will be easy.

The mistake you are making is never collecting the tools. Each time you begin again you are back to square one.

The catching point program is designed for you to begin digging the hole, rest a bit and eat, gather your strength, *and maintain your motiva-*

tion. Then dig a bit more until you get to the shovel. The difference here is, you are going to keep the shovel with you, go back and rest, eat, let some time pass. Then you are going back *to the same hole* and dig *with your shovel* until you get to the next tool, and so on. At the end you will have all the tools you need to dig a 10-by-10 hole easily, anytime you want. This is the life of the people at the catching point. They have these tools, so they just jump in and dig a new hole every time the wind changes direction or the new *Ninja Abs in 14 Days* book comes out. And you can too!

In this context, the goal will be to come out of the program with *as much as possible*. To date, you've come out with *nothing* because it's over as soon as you miss the Wednesday workout or you eat carbs. Part 2 of this book will spell out how to do this, depending on how you feel on a given day. The idea is to amass as many of these positive changes as possible. The more you accumulate, the faster you reach the catching point, and the more transformed you will be.

At the end of the program, I want *all* of you to stand with me transformed. To be ready to go on with new lives, new workouts, good feelings, and peace. This program will provide enough options so that everyone can capture these changes in ways that fit well with their individual lives, as different as they may be.

CHAPTER 3—

Becoming One of Them

Willpower won't solve the problem. Just because you want to change and put everything into making that change doesn't mean you'll make the change. It may work for a bit, but you'll get tired and stop the effort.

—Rick Warren, Author of *The Power to Change Your Life*

IVANKA TRUMP HAS MORE OPPORTUNITIES in life than you do. She does. Because of money and connections. And money. But she is just as susceptible to getting the flu and has no up-front advantage in a foot race. The point is, things like disease and sports are equalizers. There are others, like death. Things that don't discriminate based on wealth or religion or race or beauty. Three Mercedes in the garage will not help someone win a marathon or protect them from cancer. The catching point program is an equalizer. People who are able to follow the most popular, sensationalized exercise and diet regimens are different. They literally, physically, have different hormone profiles and structure that allows them to do it. Every person who picks up this book has the same fundamental anatomy and the same basic human biology and therefore has the same chance to succeed.

To date, separation between success and failure in this space has been based on misdirection. On smoke and mirrors that have caused you to waste energy on programs that weren't going to get you there. As author Geoff Colvin described in his classic book *Talent Is Overrated*, it is not blind effort or natural-born gifts that separate you from the people who have what you would like. It is *simply knowing the way* so your efforts to get there can be deliberate.[41] We will have to reorganize workout days and nurture recovery to do this, but first, let's consider the changes that will transform your body.

The changes that you accumulate between your workouts will bridge the gap between you and the successful people in fitness. They will get you to the catching point. Being attentive to, and accumulating these changes, are the specific kinds of effort necessary to transform your body to a body ready for success.

Without the catching point program, signals sent out by the brain to regular people when they stop eating are harsh, powerful, irresistible messages to stop the madness—as shown in figure 10.[6–8, 42–44] Starting on the left, the figure depicts how traditional diet changes and calorie cuts send an alarming message to the brain: we're starving! The brain then, following thousands of years of evolutionary learning, rains hell down on you until you stop it (this is the source of the feelings you have on days 2 or 3 or 4, traditionally). The catching point program aims to create happy links between the brain and clean eating *by harnessing and facilitating the positive changes that occur in between workouts*. New links mean new feelings and fewer struggles with diet and exercise, like Sally Yogapants on the right.

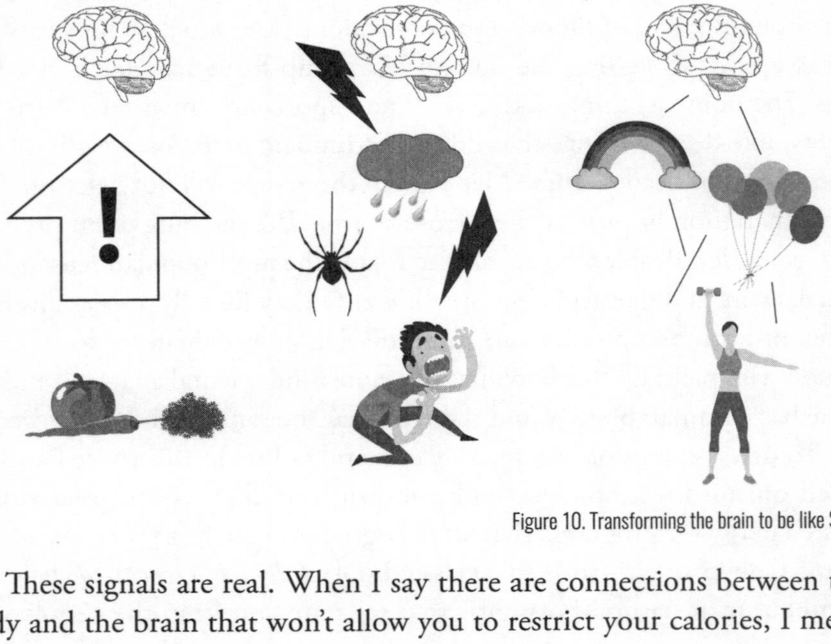

Figure 10. Transforming the brain to be like Sally.

These signals are real. When I say there are connections between the body and the brain that won't allow you to restrict your calories, I mean there are *known molecules* that have been *well described* that are accountable for people quitting their diets.[44–47] They have names. Leptin, ghrelin, GLP-1, PYY, and CCK. Bariatric surgery works because it changes the levels of these molecules.[5, 6, 44, 48] The key is resetting this system so that you feel like Sally when dieting and exercising. It can be done through surgery, through gastric artery embolization or cryovagotomy (more on these later), and on your own.

> The right combination of exercise, recovery, and supplementation will alter ghrelin levels so that long term you feel less hungry.

Ghrelin is the hunger hormone. It is produced mainly in the stomach and gets to the brain either through the bloodstream or through nerve connections—either way, it transmits the same message: "Eat!" As you can imagine, a gazillion dollars are currently being spent on developing a drug to block this hormone. So far, no dice—but these studies have revealed that bariatric surgery and gastric artery embolization decrease levels of ghrelin and people feel less hungry. Dieting, on the other hand, increases ghrelin levels. Diets do not work. But here is what is awesome: the right combination of exercise, recovery, and supplementation will alter ghrelin levels so that long term you feel less hungry.[7–9, 49]

Leptin is the fullness hormone. It is produced by fat cells and circulates in the bloodstream to tell your brain when you are full.[10, 11] In humans who overeat, this system is reset. Over time, the body starts to be resistant to leptin—again, not dissimilar to antibiotic resistance developed by bacteria that are overexposed to a given medicine. When our body sees so much leptin every day because we eat so much more than we need to survive, we develop a real resistance—and don't feel as full. Even more disturbing, the processed sugar that is added to fast foods specifically creates a need in the brain to eat. It literally addicts you in the same way nicotine addicts cigarette smokers.[50]

So, we have conditioned our bodies to need *more* leptin than usual for us to feel full. Then, once that state is established, we abruptly *drop* the leptin levels with exercise and weight loss, while at the same time increasing ghrelin.[12, 13, 51, 52] That's right, exercise and weight loss have been shown time and time again to *decrease* leptin levels and *increase* ghrelin levels, creating a miserable situation of intense hunger and food obsession. As a matter of survival, the body will prioritize food seeking. Scientists all over the world are scrambling to make a drug that will simulate leptin and make you feel full. In the meantime, we have to manage this ourselves.

> Even more disturbing, the processed sugar that is added to fast foods specifically creates a need in the brain to eat. It literally addicts you in the same way nicotine addicts cigarette smokers.

People at the catching point don't feel this because they have reconditioned their systems to need less leptin to feel full, and they don't lose crazy amounts of weight that signal to the brain they are starving. The way to join them is to continue to eat and exercise. This will modify your receptor systems to require less leptin over time without the abrupt withdrawal.[53]

To make a few comparisons, consider the power of the wired-in human sex drive or the withdrawal of a heroin addict. Both occur because of molecular signaling disruption just like how you feel when you start the diet and exercise duo of doom.

Imagine what would happen if I instituted a program to control the population, and the rules were that no one from 20 to 40 years old could have sex ever—starting Monday. What do you think the success rate would be? Do you think many humans could just shut that drive off and forget about it? Could be happy and enjoy life the same way those do who have voluntarily shut it off? Like nuns or monks? Of course not.

These urges are biological and can only be contained for limited periods of time. The same is true here. Humans can't just shut off the food-consumption urge that is wired in for our survival and expect to be successful. However, just like the nuns or monks (or whomever) who voluntarily refrain from sexual relations, the brain can be adapted to diminish that signal. Importantly, and at the risk of being repetitive, life without 4,000 calories a day, for those who are already at the catching point, is not a struggle. These people no longer receive those signals and as a result don't feel that same urge to consume *to survive* as the general population does on day 1 of a diet. So for them, it is easy!

Likewise, heroin addicts cannot just quit heroin on Monday. Again, it's not because they lack discipline or willpower; it's because their brains have become restructured to require the heroin molecule. This restructuring is a real thing! Not some made-up clinical blah blah, but a real change in molecules in the brain that can be documented.[42, 54, 55] The syndrome that heroin addicts go through when withdrawing from the drug is predictable and reproducible, and it happens every time until the body restructures its molecules to survive on less (or no) heroin. Same with food (figure 11).

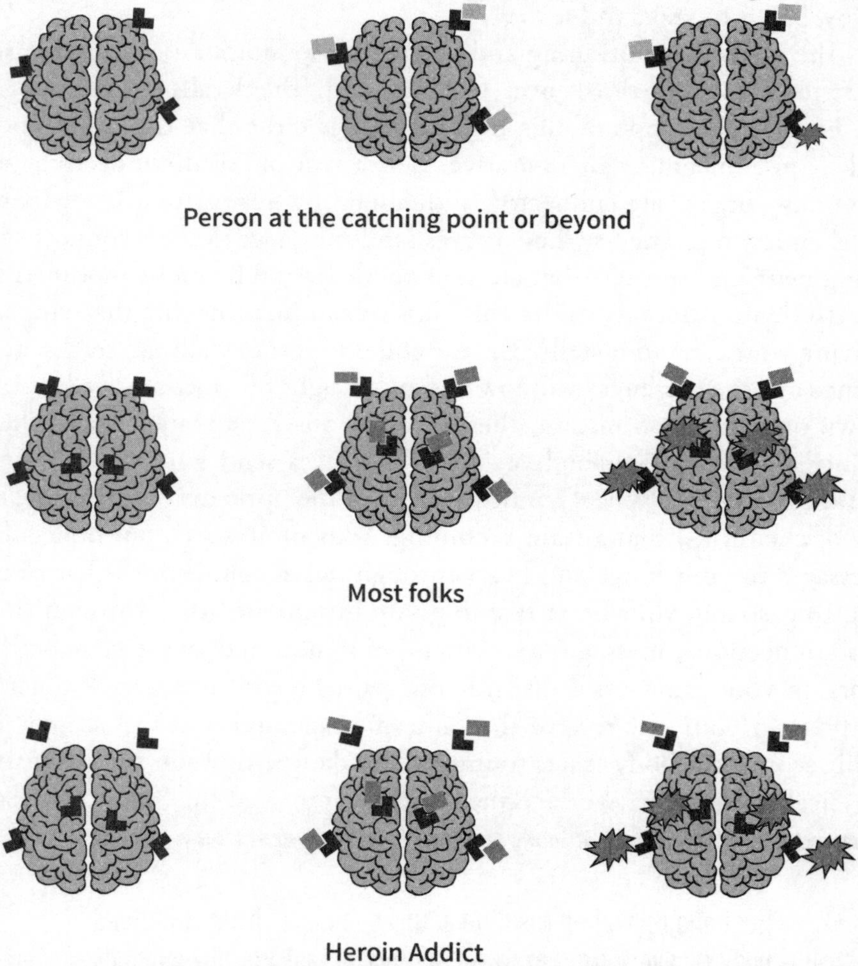

Figure 11. At baseline (column one), most folks (i.e., overeaters) are no different than heroin addicts with regard to brain molecular structure. In column two, when plenty of everything is available, everyone is happy. In column three, when food or heroin becomes sparse, the brain goes bananas sending signals from the empty receptors. The catching point person literally feels *much* less discomfort (if any) in the face of less food.

Changes in response to exercise and the right combination of nutrients—accumulated over time, in between workouts—result in different signals being sent to the brain, signals that convey to the brain that its body is *not* in danger of starving and *not* experiencing some life-threatening event against which it must defend. In fact, it is signaling that the body is getting stronger. That what is happening is good for survival, good for evolution, good for health—messages to which the brain responds with positive feedback, mediated through transmitters that cause feelings of hope, euphoria, and overall mood elevation, which are feelings that we enjoy, begin to seek, and *want*.

The idea of conditioning and changing the molecules our brains secrete to adjust behavior is over 100 years old. The details of the changes are beyond the scope of this book, but it is clear that the mind-body link is not imaginary or figurative. It is a real physical connection (all the body's organs are connected to the brain by nerves) that is mediated by chemical messengers (these nerves send messages to their connections using neurotransmitters that are well defined), and it can be modified.[53]

To demonstrate, consider this classic example: Imagine that you are driving your car and it stalls. The car glides to rest on railroad tracks. You glance out the passenger window and catch sight of a locomotive bearing down on you. In an instant, these connections are apparent—and their ability to modify your body evident. Your eyes send a message to your brain (through a physical connection called the optic nerve, using a variety of chemicals) that a train is coming. Your brain sends out molecular messages to your lungs and heart through nerve connections that cause you to gasp and your heart rate to go up instantaneously. Through similar connections, messages are sent to your skin and sweat glands. The hairs on your arms stand up and your palms begin to sweat. The nerve endings in your gut receive the same message and you feel scared. In milliseconds the body reacts to impending danger through this extensive physical-chemical network connecting the brain and the body. *This same network shuts you down when you switch to starvation on a dime.*

> Rest and relaxation result in actual chemical changes that aid body recovery from exercise, a process that literally changes a person into a different person.

Fortunately, it can also be exploited for change. The best example of this that I have seen in my career is the phenomenon of phantom pain.[56–61] Amputees experience signals from their residual limb that tell them their foot—which is no longer there—itches or hurts. Brain MRI exams of these patients have shown that their brains are organized in such a way that they really feel signals from that missing foot. The feeling is not "psychological" or "in their heads" but can be mapped using imaging as a real, reproducible phenomenon. But here is the thing: these patients' brains can be changed by changing the signals sent in from the body.[62–64] The point here is, the brain can be changed to respond differently to input—to respond differently to diet and exercise. I am not talking about your thoughts or your perception or your willpower. This is actual brain change documented on MRI and obtained through changing the input signals to the brain.

This can be used to your advantage. The brain has other functions beside survival-related blasts.[65, 66] In fact, conveniently, it works hand in hand with recovery from workouts. It has been well established that neurotransmitters sent in response to rest accelerate recovery. Conversely, signals from stressful situations such as death, work or financial issues, and marital strains slow and interrupt recovery. And, as if on cue, recovery itself results in brain changes that slowly dampen the painful response to diet over time and changes the way clean eating is viewed and experienced. This bears restating: rest and relaxation result in actual chemical changes that aid body recovery from exercise, a process that literally changes a person into a different person with different molecular structure than when they started. These microstructure changes, then, feed signals back to the brain that change its outlook on clean eating, survival, and diet—which then does away with the stress caused by diet changes so that recovery is accelerated further, and so on. The cycle feeds off itself like a snowball gaining momentum. It is kinetic (figure 12).[3]

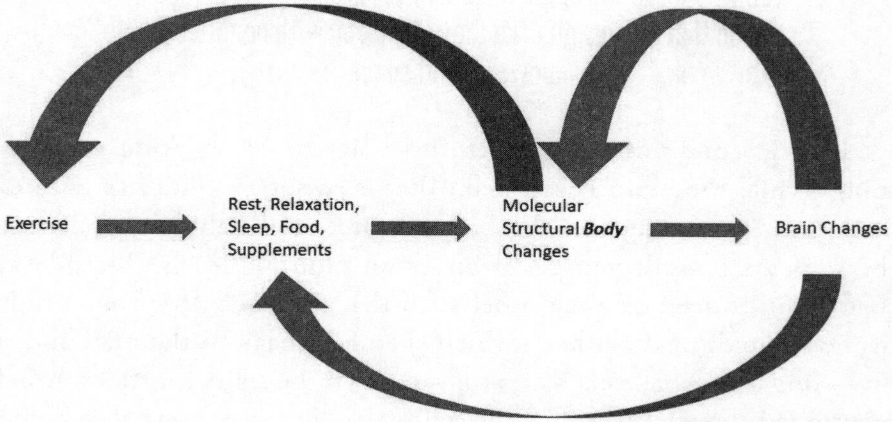

Figure 12. The healthy living feedback loop.

3 More details on kinetic change can be found in appendix 1. It gets a little dense and potentially boring, so I put it there in case you are interested.

Concentrating on accumulating changes between workouts results in the kinetic conditioning of one's heart, body, and soul *peacefully* and *without deprivation* (remember, deprivation, restriction, and stress are the senses to which the brain reacts), and the signaling pattern is reversed—the brain will actually start to signal the body *not* to eat so much and to enjoy working out. At this point (you guessed it, the catching point) your brain will be sending you signals to eat cleaner, so you will *want* to do so. You will replace that hysterical signal to eat everything in sight with one that *craves* foods lower in calories and *seeks* physical activity as a relaxant. This is how the beautiful people feel, which is why they are smiling all the time. This is also why they have *no idea* why you would ever struggle with their programs. They don't experience that same signal, so they paste you with negative labels like "weak," "no willpower," and so on. But these labels—other than maybe serving as self-fulfilling prophecies—are absolutely empty and false. Of course, you don't know how any of these lean folks would fare if they faced the same powerful signals to quit, but you aren't looking to prove that they would struggle. You are looking to reverse and extinguish your own signals—and join them.

> This is how the beautiful people feel, which is why they are smiling all the time. This is also why they have ***no idea*** why you would ever struggle with their programs. They don't experience that same signal, so they paste you with negative labels like "weak," "no willpower," and so on.

Kinetic conditioning reverses these signals by working on other things while the brain is satisfied. That is, while you are full and not panicked, you strengthen the body, create good habits, and nurture the soul. As a result you get stronger on multiple levels. These levels then begin to feed off each other such that the strength of one results in the strength of the others, which then feed back to the first, and so on—similar to a ball that starts rolling down the stairs (or the snowball mentioned above). Over time the rolling ball or large snowball becomes the dominant force, and other things follow it. For you, the body-soul-heart complex grows so strong that it becomes the dominant force, and the brain follows. Once the brain is on board, the rest is easy—you've passed through the catching point.

> You don't know how any of these lean folks would fare if they faced the same powerful signals to quit, but you aren't looking to prove that they would struggle. You are looking to reverse and extinguish your own signals—and join them.

CHAPTER 4—

Unlocking the Process

Some would rather run down and get one...I'd rather walk down and get 'em all.

— Ludacris, rapper and actor

Progress, not perfection.

— Denzel Washington as Robert McCall in *The Equalizer*

LUDACRIS WAS TALKING about being a figurative "bull" in the hip-hop industry and explaining that although some, presumably less experienced rappers would prefer to *run* down a hill and thereby gather only one "cow" (which I think in hip-hop represents a source of income), he would rather take his time, be controlled, walk down said hill, and get *all* the cows. I agree with Luda. To illustrate, consider Jane.

Jane was my coworker for many years. Jane is a bit overweight and sedentary. She has never really exercised for any significant length of time in her life, which is to say that she has limited knowledge of exercise physiology. I've watched her over the years come in on Monday after Monday declaring that "this is day 1 of my diet!" I'd watch her unpack a salad with no dressing as a snack and describe her exercise program to the girls in the break room who listened intently. She'd say how she wasn't going to eat after 6:00 p.m., how she planned to walk around the hospital with her pedometer at lunch, how her family would be "on their own" with regard to dinner during her diet, how her aunt's friend lost 80 pounds on this diet, and on and on.

One Monday it was someone's birthday and a cookie basket was delivered in their honor. Jane was stricken. The girls were giggling and eating cookies and celebrating a birthday together in the afternoon, and Jane looked like her dog had just died. I asked, "Why don't you have one? It's a special day." She didn't want to have one, because it meant the end of her program. If she ate that cookie and joined in that party, she would officially be "off her diet." It meant giving up. It meant failure. It meant restarting. Jane's focus was restriction. She believed that she could change her body by reducing calorie counts.

I am here to announce to all of the Janes (and Dicks) in the world that that way of thinking is absolutely, categorically, and unquestionably *false*. That you have not reached goals because that is not the way. I submit to every trainer, every nutritionist, every fitness expert in the world that the changes people are looking for can only occur during rest, and that a different way of thinking (a way that allows for that cookie and for a fun, enjoyable existence) is warranted to finally overcome this widespread history of repeated failures.

I submit to every trainer, every nutritionist, every fitness expert in the world that the changes people are looking for can only occur during rest, and that a different way of thinking (a way that allows for that cookie and for a fun, enjoyable existence) is warranted to finally overcome this widespread history of repeated failures.

Three overarching themes will prevail in our *new* way: *no dietary restrictions, no going backwards, and no perfection goals.* First and foremost, until the brain starts craving less or different food, don't force it. Eat what you want. Eat when you are hungry. Let the brain be in charge. Over time these signals will subtly change, and diet will quietly adjust itself without any overt effort or "willpower." During the 84 days of the changing point transformation, we aim only to include things in our diet that will aid in our recovery and rewiring, never to restrict. The program hinges on allowing and aiding your body in its change. The focus is on changing your body in a way that brings you to the catching point and evens the playing field—a process that should be enjoyable and should make you feel better.

In fact, during your pursuit of the catching point, you want to nurture and encourage the kinetic changes through dietary supplements. It will be important to *add* things to your diet in order to accelerate and facilitate recovery. Modern medical research has clearly identified foods that aid in the molecular reorganization following exercise, the changes that we seek.[33, 67–75] Also, adding these clean foods to your diet, instead of substituting, will create a positive brain-body link. New foods are introduced as soldiers for rebuilding and facilitators of adaptation—activities that the brain sees as important for survival and evolution. As a result, you begin to reverse and reorganize the signals we have been talking about. The same primitive need to survive led the brain to send you signals of depression, misery, and insatiable hunger when you substituted clean foods and cut calories because the brain associated that with starving. Now, you will be associating the same foods with rebuilding, surviving, and evolving—all things the brain is happy about. You will see, then, as time goes on how these habits will "catch" and the brain will send positive signals in response to clean eating—the kind of signals successful people are used to. The kind of signals that squash the willpower requirement.

Modern medical research has clearly identified foods that aid in the molecular reorganization following exercise, the changes that we seek.

Second, you must build safety walls to protect you from that all too well-known backward slide. Transformation occurs through recovery and rewiring, as explained in chapter 3. In order to follow the exercise programs that lead to success, your body must change and adjust along the way *on the inside.*

To understand this principle, let's expand on our hole-digging example. This time, let's say that instead of transforming from an obese person (I know, that is such an ugly-sounding label) into a rewired person at the catching point, your goal is to climb Mount Everest. If you took the same approach to fitness most people usually do, you would buy a whole bunch of mountain-climbing gear (most of which you don't know how to use), you would plan a starting day (almost always a Monday, right?), and you would spend a few weeks gearing up in your mind. Then, on the fateful "day 1" you would begin running up the mountain, straight toward the top—without breaking. Of course you are not in shape for this, and you don't get very far before you declare that you "just can't climb mountains, no matter what I try."

Now, if you employ kinetic principles of the catching point program to the same goal, it goes differently. *The key difference of this program is that at the end of your attempt, you are some distance up the mountain—not back at the bottom, planning your next attempt.* So, you begin and you get some height. Then you stop and readjust your settings, because now you are a bit farther along and the task has become that much less daunting. You set up camp, and now you are no longer at the bottom of the mountain. You stay here, eat, rest, and look around. Then, when you feel good again, you take a few more steps toward the summit. What has happened in between is that you've reset your expectations and gained strength from the initial climb. You then carefully continue on, listening to your body and mind along the way, and finding clearings and stable places to rest and camp along the way. You also realize that the air is getting thinner as you go up—something you didn't know before because even if your sprint got you up this far, you never were calm enough to observe your surroundings and listen to your body, you were just falling straight back to the beginning. Finally, you realize that you are afraid of heights, so at each new level you take time to reset your baseline and quell your fears.

The point is, at each new level you don't feel pressure to climb again the next day because your schedule says "Wednesday—5 miles up." Rather, you wait and acclimate your body *and take the journey in chunks.* And that acclimation is real. It is actual chemical and physical changes in your body's ability to tolerate thinner air and in your mind to respond calmly to new heights. Similar changes will take place in your body as you approach the catching point. Also, just as after you reach the peak of the mountain the rest of the journey is downhill, so is the remainder of the journey to your fitness goals from the catching point.

Another way to think of this is in "levels." Real changes occur in between the levels if you support them. Imagine that your journey to the catching point is represented in figure 12A, where E is the catching point (and the blue-head no-face guy is you).

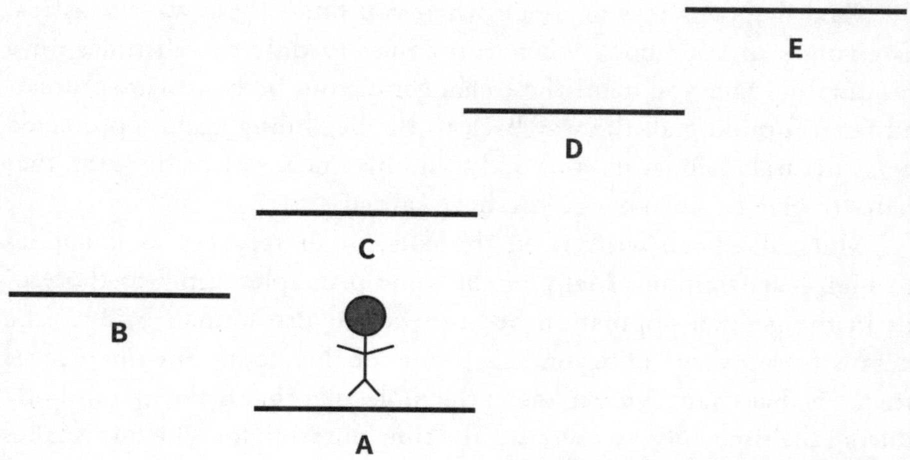

Figure 12A. The levels approach to the catching point.

As you progress up the levels, it will be critical to build walls behind you so that you never go back to A. The wall is made of physical changes you collect during rest. You aren't under any time pressure to get to the next level; *you are tasked only with not going backward.* Wall building is done through rest and diet supplements, to be detailed later. For this chapter we are focusing on what happens to your body *if* you build the walls—which are figuratively shown in figure 13.

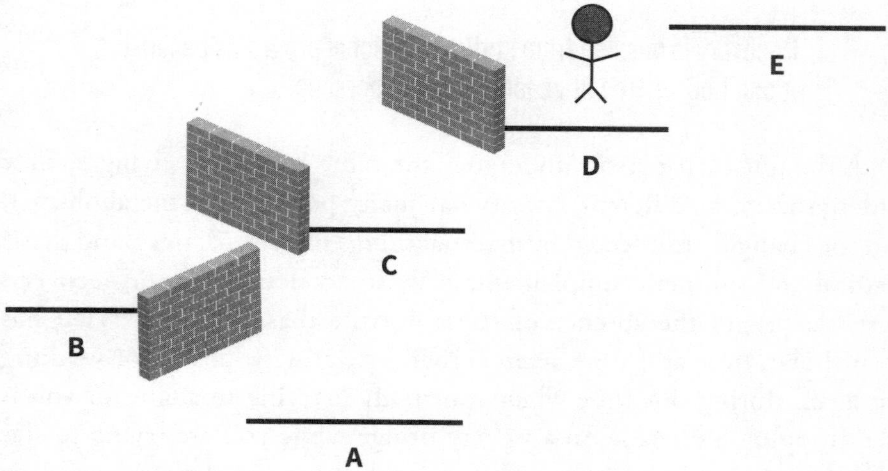

Figure 13. The walls that protect you from backsliding.

What happens to your body when you build these walls is as real as changes in your body when you adjust to different altitudes on a mountain. Once you make these changes in your body, you are protected from tumbling all the way back to the beginning again—protected by structural changes in your body, and by a new way of thinking that hates to give up any change you have earned.

Much has been written on the concept of recovery as it applies to high-level training. Many of the same principles apply to those of us in the general population because we are also human beings. The details of recovery are beyond the scope of this book, but the general theme is that changes are made in the molecules that make up our body during the time *after* we exercise. The time duration for which this takes place is variable, depending on the person in question, the exercise, and what else is happening during the recovery period. Under ideal circumstances, your body reorganizes its molecular structure just a bit after every workout for 24 to 36 hours. This is critical to our program because each time this happens, a few bricks are added to your wall. Literally, the makeup of your lungs, heart, and muscles changes, and as a result you start changing into a different person. Your body sends telltale signals that it is undergoing this process, and you must recognize and manage them.

> Recovery is missing from static, traditional programs because it can't be written in generically. It is personal....

Although each person undergoes the same biological changes, they undergo them at different rates (what many people call "metabolism"), and the changes are affected by external things like sleep, stress, and diet.[4] Natural and synthetic supplements exist to accelerate and aid recovery. Rest, sleep, and the absence of stress nurture these changes. What has been shown time and time again is that restricting your diet or working out again during this time when your body is trying to adapt for you is like dropping a grenade on a rickety bridge while you are trying to stabilize it. You have to let the stabilization happen, let the strengthening progress from the inside out.

4 "Stress" here refers to traditional stress from work, bills, kids, spouses, and so on.

So far we have learned the following:

1. The major difference between you and the people who can successfully follow diet and exercise programs is the structure of your body deep down, on the inside.

2. In order to make the necessary micro changes, you must allow yourself to benefit from the in-between days and even nurture this process.

3. Your body will send you signals that it is changing, and you must react accordingly.

4. A major reason for failure with all these programs for untrained people like Jane is that they never recover. They either sprint straight up the mountain and quit, or—even if they follow the program to the letter—skip the recovery and never change, so they are always at the beginning.

Recovery is missing from static, traditional programs because it can't be written in generically. It is personal and varies for each one of us. As a result, you must learn to manage it yourself and accept that following these signals means abandoning the "perfect attendance" goal you set when you try to follow programs marketed for the masses. This is the substance of the catching point program.

CHAPTER 5—
Building Walls

Nothing breeds success like success.

—Anonymous

WE KNOW FROM EXPERIENCE that it's not likely we will just wake up one day and be successful with a diet. It's like trying to hold your breath. At some point you just have to give up. The key is to prevent the "white knuckle" days. To get something that gives you an edge. To prepare your body in such a way that it doesn't send you overwhelming "eat and quit" messages that you feel like you have to resist. The critical element that has been missing for you so far is to prevent those days, to take the focus off that part of it and follow a map that takes you around those obstacles to your destination.

The catching point program seeks to increase your exercise capacity so you don't feel that way when the diet starts. You want to accumulate changes that will make you comfortable during a diet so you can be successful. To get there, to benefit from these changes, we introduced two overarching principles to understand: no diet restrictions, and no going backward.

We talked a bit about not restricting diet and will revisit that topic again later. In this chapter, we will expand on the principle of not going backward, of building those safety walls. In order to do so, you will employ flexibility with the workouts, diet supplements, soul shaping, and rest to provide a safety net/barricade when you start to feel in the pits.

The concepts behind wall building are broadly separated into four categories: range, no restart, the slowly moving cliff, and do no harm.

Range

Boxers define range as the distance from their opponent they can stand without getting hit. If they misjudge or disregard range, they are in danger of being knocked out of the fight. Same here. If you get too crazy with your diet or too stringent with your workout schedule because you misjudge or ignore your body's signals, you are in danger of being knocked out of this fight, the fight to change your body. It is important that you *get as much done as possible* during this program—and to do so will require several sidesteps and rest stops. Your goal is to stay out of striking distance from the quit monster. If you start to feel like you are too tired, less motivated, distracted, or hungry, you are in range of the quit monster and you need to back off a bit. We aren't looking to be heroes here, we are just trying not to get knocked out.

No Restart (and the "Do Nothing" Clause)

You want to progress and build walls on your days off. As a result, there is no value to starting over. Starting over leads to repeating the day 1 or day 2 workouts 10,000 times, which isn't worth jack crap. Here, if you can't get to the tasks for a week or three, you just pick up where you left off. This is important and worth stressing. You are interested in reaching a point of transformation that will allow you to achieve your goals through a follow-up, standard diet and exercise program—a point you likely have been unable to reach so far through those same standard programs. In order to get to this point, the catching point, you need to stay after these tasks and not start over, regardless of how many times you get derailed.

Once the catching point program is initiated, *there is no restarting and no quitting*. This is a step-wise change in your body's signals, and it cannot be "reset" because of the wall behind you. You will see as we go on that these actions are to be incorporated into real life, with all of its emotions, unexpected occurrences, busyness, changing deadlines, and so forth. This is reality based. This is not a video game that you can start over if you don't like the way the opening scenes go. There will be no reason to start over or quit, because there is no failure, there is only chunky progress.[5] Also the program is not uncomfortable, and it is repeatable—depending on what level of fitness you are after. It consists of many buckets of tasks available for completion when you feel ready.

We will talk more about the specific options of the program in the second half of the book. For now, though, the idea of chunky process should be expanded upon. Imagine that you are a collector of rare coins, and you hope to one day have a collection of all of a certain series of coins. They are hard to come by, so you can't just walk into a store and buy the whole set. What you would do, then, is always keep the idea of your collection in the back of your mind and collect coins "in chunks" as the opportunities presented themselves. For example, if you are on a vacation, you might take a day to travel to a certain location that is known to have coins of your type and buy a few. Conversely, if you had two busy days at work, you wouldn't worry about the coins, but you *would* keep the coins you have collected in a safe place. You would not say, "Well, I had two busy days at work and I couldn't add to my coin collection, so I'm going to throw all my coins out and start over." You would add to your collection in chunks, as your life allowed.

Same thing here. You will pull from the program's options as life allows and accumulate changes in the same way you accumulated coins in this example. Reflect at the end of the week on what you have done, and be glad you are that much closer to your dreams, to completing your coin collection. Same same.

Similarly, consider the typical rags-to-riches story. It goes something like this:

> I saw all those rich men and women in their fancy cars going into those big office buildings. I dreamt I could do it, I worked hard, I saved along the way, kept my nose to the grindstone, and the breaks started coming. I capitalized on this or that break, continued to work hard, and it led to X.

The hero of our story made their way in chunks. They stayed after it. The alternative story would maybe go like this:

5 That is, progress in chunks. Not chunky's progress—that would not be nice.

> I saw all those rich men and women in their fancy cars going into those big office buildings. I dreamt I could do it, I worked hard, then one day it didn't go well so I quit the whole thing and started over.

The moral is, don't quit—that won't end in a penthouse interview in New York City. People who succeed take a few lumps, have a few down days, take a few days off, *and then they keep going.*

To be clear, though—I'm not saying push through the tough times. I'm saying come back to where you left off *after* the tough times. This is where the "do nothing" clause comes in to play. Each time you start to feel that darkness creep in, vow to do nothing for 24 hours. Don't make any decisions one way or the other, don't work out, don't recover, don't even think about the program. Just literally stop in your tracks and do nothing. After 24 hours, return to the program and decide what you want to do. You can certainly swap in a day off or a recovery massage at that point (see chapter 10), but the real value will be that *you are still on board.* Got that? Good. Now let's start considering what leads to the fall in the first place.

The Slowly Moving Cliff

Related to no restart is the idea of our slowly moving cliff. (I suppose we could even tie this into the canyon romance from chapter 1 if we really reach.) Anyway, the transformation to the catching point through this program should be viewed as walking toward a cliff that is slowly moving away from you. If you go faster than the cliff is moving, you end up like Wile E. Coyote in the classic Looney Tunes cartoon. The cliff moves slowly away as you walk. As a result, if you go too fast (i.e., do too much, as you most certainly would embarking on a brand-new exercise program), you fall off.

Now, in traditional programs this marks the end, the give-up day—after which you restart the cycle. In the catching point program, though, this is not the case. When you sense that you have taken on too much, that you don't feel like being on a program anymore, that you are tired, less motivated, whatever, you slow down or stop and let the cliff move ahead of you. This is in stark contrast to what you are used to, which is the start-over cycle described multiple times above.

During this transformation, it is imperative that you stop and slow down every time you feel the urge. It only matters that you progress; it does not matter when. To translate this into actual exercise terms, it is better to take two weeks off and come back in at workout 3 than to quit and restart in a week at workout 1. The reason for this is that the workouts accomplish progressively more, so that coming in and doing workout 10 is worth ten times as much with regard to metabolism, air exchange, calorie burning, and so on than workout 1. Repeating a workout 1 over and over because of habitual "do-overs" is silly. No do-overs.

Signs that you are approaching the fall include waning interest in the program, the desire to "just start over another day," fatigue, and mood change. More on this later, but suffice it to say, this program is not supposed to be unpleasant. *If you feel bad, you are too close to the cliff.*

This matters because human beings are not built to constantly move forward toward any goal. Anytime we identify something as a goal and start toward it, we can only continue toward it for a certain amount of time at once. For example, if we decided it would be useful to get to the next state on foot and set out at a full sprint toward said state, we would quickly run out of energy, at which point we would be in danger of giving up. I mean, we emptied our tank and probably only went 200 yards and would still have miles to go. Very discouraging.

On the other hand, if we embraced the idea that *the important thing is to get as far as possible*, then we would start out walking. In fact, it is likely that we would take the time to pack a bag with water and snacks and money, and maybe a map. We would make sure we had durable shoes and the right clothes. And maybe a hat and sunglasses for the Florida-to-Georgia trip. Or snow boots for the Illinois-to-Ohio trip. Then we would begin slowly on the right track—focused on getting as far as possible. We would walk a comfortable distance, then rest, realizing that this was going to take time and that emptying our tank one day to get an extra half mile probably wouldn't be worth it when we had 200 miles to go. If we developed a blister on our foot we would address it, not "push through it," but we would also not give up because of it. If our focus is longer term, then we could take two days and let it heal. Spend time wrapping it up so it didn't hurt. When the focus is getting in as many miles as possible, we will have to pace ourselves to get it done—and how that translates is important.

Your body will tell you when you need to break. No schedule, no program, no written routine can anticipate how an individual's body will react to stress.[6] The analogy of the slowly moving cliff is meant to make the point that you cannot start at a sprint on "day 1" or you will end up like Wile E., but it is also meant to make the point that this will be a "stop and go" program. You will need to stop for days at a time and know that that's OK. The cliff is moving slowly away so when you take days off, you are making yourself safe. You are ensuring that you don't run off the cliff. The traditional A-to-B programs (see chapter 1) are unreasonable because if on day 5 your body and mind need rest, but the program says to cook seaweed and rice for dinner and do 60 minutes on the exercise machine, you are out! Screw it! And a few more months go by before you try it again.

To reach the catching point, the important thing is to keep progressing. If it were written like a traditional exercise program (which it is not), that would mean that if on day 5 you feel like you are going off the cliff, you sit down and rest and let the cliff move away. When you feel safe again that you aren't going to fall off, you slowly rise and it would still be day 5. So if it takes 90 days to complete a 15-day program, it doesn't matter, because you still get the benefits of a 15-day program, which puts you that much further ahead. As long as it gets done at some point without falling off the cliff is all that matters, because when you fall off the cliff you give up and leave with nothing, as opposed to not falling off the cliff and having 15 days of solid work done at the 90-day point. These numbers are made up, of course, but the point is, the important thing for reaching the catching point is to be aware of how close to the cliff you are getting (range) and that there is no restart here, only a list of things to get done over time.

> ...if it takes 90 days to complete a 15-day program, it doesn't matter, because you get the benefits of a 15-day program, which puts you that much further ahead.

Do No Harm

OK, this one is important. I mean, they are all important, but this one maybe should have been Rule #1. The entire premise of this program is to transform your body in between workouts so that you will be successful in the future. If, in between workouts, you do harm, then you are dead in the water.

6 "Stress" in this context means a change in routine, not mental stress like bills or mothers-in-law or people giving you the finger in traffic.

That means no getting drunk. And no sleep deprivation. The program itself is pretty flexible and fail-safe as a whole, but these two things are veritable land mines we have to be careful of. Getting drunk during the 90 days or going on a stretch with inadequate sleep is like tipping the new level you've reached so you slide under the wall you've built, as in figure 15. To build off our previous analogy, it will be like slipping on rocks and sliding back down the mountain you've been so carefully climbing and smashing your face on the way down.

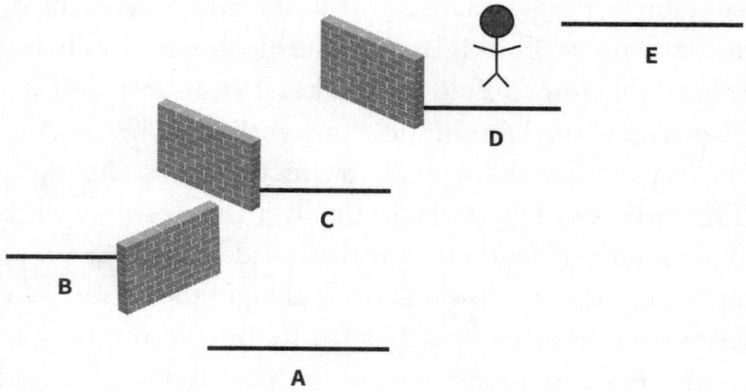

Remember this figure? This is you in the Catching Point Program. Secure and cozy with your safety wall built. You could rest here for days, weeks even–then make your way up to E.

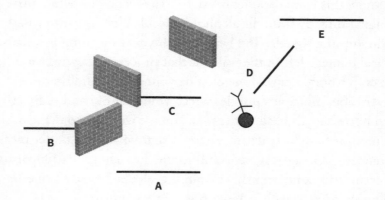

This is the effect of alcohol or sleep deprivation on the Catching Point progress.

Figure 15

The reason for this is as follows. Resting on the D platform will aid in recovery. Even if you rest beyond the time it takes your body to recover (because you've eaten protein, taken the right vitamins, avoided stress, etc.—more on this soon), you've made long-term changes to your body that are stable. Stable means *the changes will be there when you come back to work out again*, unless you actively do something to damage your body.

Without getting too scientific, alcohol is a molecule that damages cells. You are spending all this time and effort to reorganize your molecules into a stable, strong, sustainable scaffold, and to send the message to your brain that your scaffold is sturdy. The alcohol molecule is like a termite that chews on your scaffold and makes it weak and, as if that weren't enough, also targets the communications with your brain. Alcohol specifically blocks processes that you are trying to harness during recovery.[76] It blocks the synthesis of glycogen in the liver (the reason we mix protein and Gatorade after our workouts, as discussed in chapter 9), accelerates the inflammatory response toward auto-damage (the reason we engage in active recovery), decreases blood flow to the recovering muscles, blocks anabolic hormones (the reason we are so crazy about sleep and food in recovery), and shifts metabolism toward fat storage and muscle wasting (do I really need to comment on that one?), and the alcohol molecule will literally blend in and damage your new neural connections and blur them into crapsville.

You know this from experience, right? The feeling of being buzzed or drunk follows directly from the alcohol molecule blending into your brain and fuzzing up the signals. The headache the next morning is because of the physical damage left in the wake of that process. Likewise, your body feels like crap from damage done outside your brain. And that is just one bout. Over time, multiple episodes wreck your scaffold and redirect your brain and nerve signals back to the pits. You are working to make positive changes in your body's structure, changes that will occur under pleasant circumstances—during rest, relaxation, and low stress. Participating in this program and concurrently consuming alcohol beyond one or two drinks a week is like stacking paper boxes in a windstorm.

Likewise, sleep is what we call an anabolic process. It is the same anabolic associated with illegal performance-enhancing drugs. Right, performance *enhancing*. It is our intention to use this natural anabolic process to our advantage for recovery and change.

The flipside of that is an ugly word spelled c-a-t-a-bolic. Catabolism is body breakdown. It is the exact opposite of what we want. Any stretch of sleep deprivation will tip your platform by breaking down the scaffold you are building. And to neatly tie this preachy-sounding section up, alcohol screws up your sleep. So build the scaffold over time: build a little on Monday, a little next Thursday, and so on, and it will still be there so you can build upon it when you return. Don't do anything to destroy or weaken it. It won't wither on its own, so you can feel safe that it will be stable and secure. Do no harm.

PART 2:

Building Your Program

CHAPTER 6—

Stay Full

Everybody has a plan until they get punched in the face.

— Mike Tyson, world heavyweight boxing champion

MR. TYSON SO ELOQUENTLY captured the essence of our diet failures in his famous quote above. The plans themselves seem great on paper. In fact, they are great. In the split second we get an unexpected assault from our brain in the name of survival, though, our plan is out the window. It's like getting punched in the face. Then we default to the spelling bee plan: miss one word (or miss one workout, have one "bad" meal) and we're out. "Undoable. U-N-D- Uh…crap, I'm out. I'll try a different spelling bee in a few weeks."

This phenomenon is so common I am betting each of you has experienced it many times, and know many others who have as well. This response is real, as described in chapter 3—and powerful. It is mediated by molecules that act on your brain, the same molecules that tell you to sleep, procreate, and protect yourself. Trying to beat that is futile.

The solution can be illustrated through a principle I call "the alpha day." A colleague of mine was discussing his newest diet while we were away on business. It sounded pretty typical, pretty solid on paper, and I told him so. Well, we returned to our hotel in the late evening of the second day of our trip (third day of his diet). As we made our way toward the elevators, we passed an automated food dispenser that, amongst other things, contained Hot Pockets. My colleague, Darvon is his name, explained to me that he was starving since he had been working out more than usual and was dying for a Hot Pocket. With drawn eyes he reported, "I have to have a Hot Pocket, I am so hungry. But what is the point, then?" I asked him to clarify. He replied, "What is the point of all this working out and sacrifice if I'm just going to eat this Hot Pocket anyway?"

Darvon was experiencing the ever-so-common "punch in the face." As mentioned several times so far, those at or beyond the catching point don't feel this same urge. Their brains have adapted to enjoy the idea of eating clean. Most of us can't get there, though, because the most powerful force working against people trying to change their fitness level is hunger. *So how can you survive this onslaught long enough to transform your body and mind so that you will enjoy eating clean?* By staying full. By understanding the concept of the alpha day. Let's see how this plays out.

I bought Darvon a Hot Pocket, told him to enjoy it—with a Coke to drink—and I scratched out the concept of the alpha day on a sheet of scrap paper (figure 16). I have also reproduced the scrap paper in table form for purposes of this explanation. The way you survive these transformation programs long enough for the idea to "catch," and your brains to adjust, is by eating the Hot Pocket when you are hungry. This accomplishes a few things. First and most importantly, it keeps you on your program. You wake up the next day and you don't feel quite as miserable or guilty, so you keep on keeping on. By doing this, you win in the long run because you outlast the onslaught and things get easier. I promise you, things are so much easier on the other side of day 30, and they are effortless on the other side of day 90.

> The way you survive these transformation programs long enough for the idea to "catch," and your brains to adjust, is by eating the Hot Pocket when you are hungry...I promise you, things are so much easier on the other side of day 30, and they are effortless on the other side of day 90.

Also, for the calorie counters, fixating on and torturing yourself over that Hot Pocket is like worrying that someone spilled a Dixie cup of water into the pool you are emptying. In the figure and table, day alpha was Darvon's day. He had consumed 1,500 calories to that point in the day and had worked out, which probably put him at a net of 1,300 calories. (No wonder he was starving!) If he doesn't eat the Hot Pocket, he goes to bed at 1,300. If he does, plus the Coke, he goes to bed at 1,800. When he is not on a diet, his typical intake is 2,500 calories a day. In addition to not chucking the whole diet—which again, is the most important benefit to eating this snack—he doesn't really alter his 90-day calorie reduction anyway. If Darvon takes in 1,300 calories a day for 90 days, which I guarantee is not doable, he will take in 117,000 calories: all gamma days from the figure = a 48 percent reduction in calorie intake. If he eats Hot Pocket and Coke snacks half the days he is on the program in order to keep his sanity and remain engaged, he will take in 139,500: half alpha days = a 38 percent reduction in calorie intake, compared to baseline. That's a 10 percent difference in calorie intake if you snack on Hot Pockets and Cokes half the time! And to think how many programs were quit and how many failures accumulated over a measly 10 percent difference!

If you get that, then here are some of the most important lines in the book: Because you ate those Hot Pockets and drank those Cokes, you were able to stay on the program to the end. And during that time, you did workouts you would not have done (thereby burning calories) and you increased your exercise capacity so you could do more valuable workouts now (more on this later). And you will have *more than surpassed* that 10 percent while at the same time adopting a new way of thinking—and changing your life.

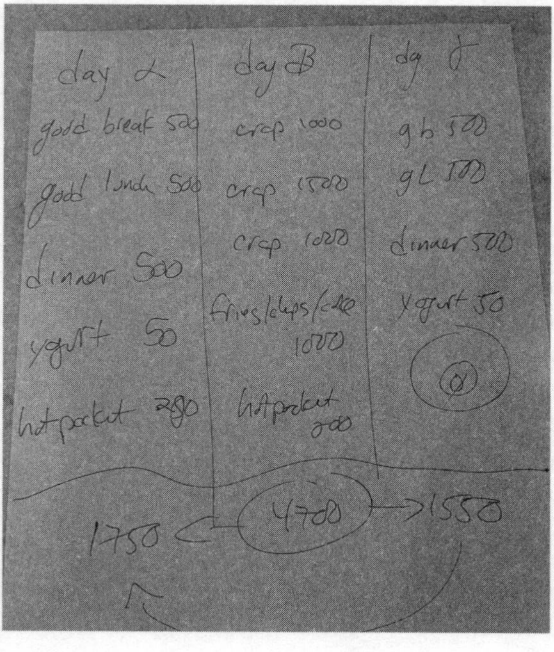

Figure 16. The actual, original alpha day explanation. It has since evolved a bit, but the core of the principle remains the same.

Day		⊠	⊠
	Breakfast 500 calories	Breakfast 500 calories	Breakfast 500 calories
	Lunch 500 calories	Lunch 600 calories	Lunch 500 calories
	Dinner 500 calories	Dinner 1,000 calories	Dinner 500 calories
	Workout –200 calories	Snack 400 calories	Workout –200 calories
	Hot Pocket and Coke Snack 500 calories		
Total	1,800	2,500	1,300
90-day total	162,000	225,000	117,000
⊠ -	63,000	0	108,000
With half ⊠ days	139,500		
⊠ -	85,500		

The alpha day principle. The difference between a textbook ▯ day and the proposed sanity-keeping ▯ day really doesn't add up to a significant difference in the grand scheme of things (see highlighted boxes), yet thousands of diets are abandoned over scenarios like the one Darvon faced every year.

So for 84 days, stay full. Stay full so (1) you don't quit and (2) you rewire your brain to crave exercise so that (3) it will start to send different signals (fun, happy signals) in response to lean eating and exercise. During this transformation, the brain will be coaxed to "get on board." You will extinguish that horrible, miserable reaction to clean eating. As explained earlier, the people who are successful with regard to fitness and diet do not feel that same overwhelming urge to eat and "go off the wagon." Rather, their brains send a positive signal out that makes them feel good about what they are doing. *So the first, and most important, step toward transformation is keeping the brain happy and calm* while you make other changes to your body that will ultimately allow you to exercise and diet like the stars. This means that during your change, while you follow the instructions in this book to get you to the catching point, there will be no diet restrictions. Later, when you have reprogrammed the brain a bit and can make changes in your diet without discomfort, we can talk more about clean eating. But for now, no diet restrictions.

Remember, it's called "the catching point" because when you put these principles in motion, over time you will start to safely move right on the figures to the corner of the triangle (chapter 1). You will stay strong and sneak along the line toward the right. At some point you will begin to *want* to exercise and eat clean, not as a means to an end, but because you literally want to do it because you enjoy it and it makes you feel *good*. The lifestyle will "catch on," with almost no effort from you—you will barely even notice it.

Afterburn

While you are feeling full and still motivated to change and not really sacrificing any significant amount of calories anyway, other critical changes are happening that will close the space between you and those people beyond the catching point. In addition to establishing the capacity to handle the mainstream fitness stuff, the restructuring of your body will also result in a calorie-burning machine *independent of exercise*.[77–80] This is a well-known phenomenon to athletes and fitness folks as well—and, to my most pleasant surprise, to Dr. Oz.

> We will keep real-time track of your changing metabolic rate based on values of the workouts, recoveries, and rest you accumulate.

Wrestlers call it the "afterburn." They work out at very high levels for many months at a super-intense pace. Typically, during the months immediately following the season, wrestlers will go crazy eating pizza and ice cream and soda and all the other things from which they have abstained during their season. The thing is, they don't gain weight during this time. Why? Because their bodies have adapted to efficiently burn what comes in. This is the most extreme example of the underlying body changes we are trying to achieve, of course, but the principle is the same. As a bonus to increasing your exercise capacity and keeping your fire lit, your basal metabolic rate (again, the way your body handles the food you eat) will also improve. You will keep real-time track of your changing metabolic rate based on the values of the workouts, recoveries, and rest you accumulate.

While researching the scientific literature for this book, I came across an article online entitled, "Dr. Oz: Fast metabolism plan with two splurge days and healthy fat days."[81] Knowing the power over the public the great Dr. Oz has, I couldn't resist reading this piece. The plan was written as advice on how to negotiate upcoming holidays, to in fact embrace opportunity in the pending days of increased caloric intake. Without repeating all the details here, it is worth pointing out that contained in this article was the most brilliant of lines, which reads as follows: "During the week, you'll be able to switch days if you want to, as long as you get all seven things on all seven days." So, Dr. Oz—being Dr. Oz—essentially captured the essence of this entire book in one line probably as an afterthought (sort of frustrating to the guy who spent 10,000 hours writing said book, but hey, whaddya gonna do…). The point is, just like pending holidays, life itself and the feedback from your body following exercise will necessitate that you be flexible with your schedule and that you eat (called "splurge days" in Dr. Oz's article) in order to stay engaged and get all the things done that will allow you to increase your exercise capacity, change your basal metabolic rate, *and transform.*

20 Minutes, Pain Meds, the Doctor's Lounge, and Metamucil

For those of you who just cannot ignore eating, or for those of you who get to the eighth workout and beyond (discussed later), here are some quasi-advanced tips and tricks. The body is programmed to shut down eating at some point, right? If not, you would just eat and eat and eat and never stop. The body senses that you have eaten through signals sent back to the brain during eating.[82,83] In order to capture and redirect these signals to your advantage, give it 20 minutes. When you sit down to eat a meal, eat half. Then, go do something else for 20 minutes. Then, come back and eat the other half. This does three things:

1. In keeping with the theme of this chapter, it will make you feel fuller. You can eat the same amount ultimately, but it will take closer to an hour—which will trick your brain into thinking you are fuller than you really are.

2. It will train your body to send signals that you are full sooner than they do now, so going forward in the long run you will feel less hungry following less food.

3. It will dampen the drive to overeat. I realize that this advice flies a bit in the face of the "stay full" mantra, so feel free to ignore it for now. I include it because I know that overall this book and its approach are unconventional and you may need a more traditional nugget to make you feel safe and because shortly into the program you are going to feel like doing more.

Consider what you do when you have a headache, or twist your ankle, or have heartburn. You take a pain medication or a TUMS, and you wait 20 minutes. You don't sit there and throw down aspirin for 20 straight minutes until your headache goes away or you die from liver failure—you wait 20 minutes and then you take another if you still have a headache. Same with TUMS or your ankle. Same here. Take the dose of food, then wait 20 minutes to see if your hunger goes away. If it's still there after that time, take some more until you feel better. It will end in 4 aspirin and probably headache relief as opposed to 40 aspirin and an emergency room visit.

Similarly, the Metamucil trick works. That is, if you can tolerate drinking Metamucil after the 20-minute break from eating, it will work even better. One tablespoon of fiber (any commercial or generic brand will work) with a large glass of water will begin the feedback cycle early. It will secure the effect of this approach by sending signals early and giving you a head start.

Finally, the doctor's lounge trick. Several times in my life when I've been out of money, I found that there is free coffee and food in the doctor's lounge. Of course the best thing for anyone to do is to pack a healthy lunch—peanut butter sandwiches, an apple, and so forth. I hate packing lunches and work at several different places, so I often found myself during the day with no food, no money, and only that doctor's lounge option. For some time I just had coffee instead of food, which isn't a terrible, terrible idea—but by the time I got home I would be pushing the kids out of the way to get to my dinner (and theirs if they were too slow).

During my catching point period—described in chapter 11—I thought I should somehow try to derail this ravenous dinner thing. So even though I didn't particularly care for any of the food in the doctor's lounge, I ate it anyway. Literally ate something that wasn't really healthy or even tasted good to me. I ate it *purposefully* in order to dampen the crazy, nuts, wild eating frenzy that was my arrival home in the evening. And it worked.

So stay full. If you feel like using these tips/tricks, please do. If not, no worries—it's gravy. Onward.

CHAPTER 7—

Create Space

A PROFESSOR ONCE FILLED a glass bucket with rocks and asked his class, "Is this bucket full?" Next, he dropped in handfuls of pebbles that filled the space between the rocks and asked, "How about now?" Then he poured in sand, which filled the spaces between the pebbles. "What about now?" Finally he allowed water to drip in, which intercalated between the sand granules. "Now?" he asked....

Below is a typical "30 day" program available on websites, in books, and anywhere else one looks for fitness advice. There is no reasonable person who will say that at the end of these 30 days, if you complete the 20 exercise intervals of the program you will not have burned a lot of calories. So, from the traditional standpoint, this is solid. (Not surprisingly, you are probably considering trying this, huh? Ugh...please read on.)

If it were possible to stick to this program, you would certainly glean the benefits of burning calories on those days, through those exercises, and no doubt from additional intake restrictions. *But* you can't do it because there is no in-between room for your body to change, so it never catches. People who are successful with diet, exercise, and wellness don't get there because they burned 250 calories on the treadmill; they *maintain* by doing that because their insides are already changed. You have a different task (different than maintaining—you are looking to change). Let's begin.

	Sunday	Monday	Tuesday	Wednesday	Thursday	Friday	Saturday
Week 1	**1.** Low-impact stretching, 20 minutes	**2.** Jog for 15 minutes	**3.** Cross-training, 10 minutes	Rest	**4.** Abs and strength training, 30 minutes	**5.** Interval training	Rest
Week 2	**6.** Uphill jog, 15 minutes	**7.** Aerobic conditioning, 20 minutes	**8.** Abs and strength training	Rest	**9.** Stretching, swimming for 30 minutes	**10.** Interval training	Rest
Week 3	**11.** Abs and strength training, 60 minutes	**12.** Interval training on track	**13.** Cross-training, 30 minutes	Rest	**14.** Belly burners and tire swings	**15.** Spinning class, 45 minutes	Rest
Week 4	**16.** Belly burners and strength training, 60 minutes	**17.** Calf raises and breadbasket weaving	**18.** Jog for 60 minutes	Rest	**19.** Interval training	**20.** Strength squats and neck raises, 50 minutes	Rest

Let's modify this table from the standpoint of the catching point. The above program is most certainly written by someone familiar with exercise to the right of the catching point (see chapter 1) and for the same kind of people. We can change it, though, to illustrate how *you* intend to get to *your* goals. As mentioned, the exercise program as written will certainly be effective. The problem, of course, is that no one will do it, and by Tuesday of week 1 most will have given up. The point of this chapter is that when someone gives up on Tuesday of week 1, it's not the calorie burns from the rest of the missed workouts that really matters—it's the inner change that would take place in between if someday you did workout 2 *when you were ready.* The real loss is that if you could finish this program at your own pace, the signals that your brain sends would begin to change. If by some miracle you got to the second 30 days, *you would feel different*, and that change would feed your momentum and the struggle that you felt on day 1 would begin to disappear. What you are really missing when you forego this program is the chance to transform from the inside out. It's not the workouts that matter; it's the inner change in between.

Let's look at this table from the catching point perspective. Over three months, here is what most people from the general population typically get done using the "start over" method (and you can imagine the same thing over six months, a year, two years….)

	Sunday	Monday	Tuesday	Wednesday	Thursday	Friday	Saturday
Week 1	**1.** Low-impact stretching, 20 minutes	**2.** Jog for 15 minutes	**3.** Cross-training, 10 minutes	Rest			
Week 2							
Week 3							
Week 4							
Week 1	**1.** Low-impact stretching, 20 minutes	**2.** Jog for 15 minutes	**3.** Cross-training, 10 minutes	Rest	**4.** Abs and strength training, 30 minutes	**5.** Interval training	Rest
Week 2							
Week 3							
Week 4							
Week 1	**1.** Low-impact stretching, 20 minutes	**2.** Jog for 15 minutes					
Week 2							
Week 3							
Week 4							

And again, it is true that for whomever these 30 days represent, they miss out on the calorie burns from the workouts—but that is not the real issue! Look, if on average the calories burned for these workouts was 300, then you would have burned approximately 18,000 calories over the month if you followed it to the letter.[7] Quitting the program a few days in and restarting every time resulted in a total of 10 workouts getting done over the 90-day period and a 3,000-calorie burn. *Of course you burn less, but the point is at that point you are still stuck at square one!* You are no better off from a capacity standpoint than you were three months ago. The difference of 16,000 calories is not your problem; it's that over *the next* three months your potential is still maxed out at 3,000 calories, and the three months after that, and so on. Whereas if somehow you did 10 workouts, burned 3,000 calories, *and got to the catching point*, you could look forward to burning 30,000 calories in the coming three months! And then mixing it up after that and getting ripped, and so forth. In order to overcome this cycle, you have to get to the point where you can look at this program and realistically plan to follow it, and in order to do that you need to benefit from the in-between magic.

7 This is an estimation to make a point; it could be any average number. Whether it's 1,100, or 1 million, the point would be the same.

> Whereas if somehow you did 10 workouts, burned 3,000 calories, *and got to the catching point*, you could look forward to burning 30,000 calories in the coming three months!

Now let's change the way you react when you start to feel like quitting. By the way, this feeling will already be less because you aren't starving, but nevertheless some urge to quit will present itself for various reasons. Instead of bailing and starting over weeks down the road, let's try a different approach. When you quit and start over, you go through this depression-like stage, then you begin to look a bit at exercise programs again, then you "set a day," spend time laying out the undoable program, and then begin again. When pursuing the catching point, you will not restart (chapter 5), so there is no need to waste all that time. If you miss workout 3, it's not over—you take a few days and then knock out workout 3. Depending on the days following that and how you feel, you get to workout 4. You don't care about keeping a schedule; you care about changing internally—even if it means 20 workouts in 84 days.

Here is why: consider the same 90 days, but using the no restart principle. It will look something like this.

	Sunday	Monday	Tuesday	Wednesday	Thursday	Friday	Saturday
Week 1	**1.** Low-impact stretching, 20 minutes	**2.** Jog for 15 minutes	**3.** Cross-training, 10 minutes	Rest			
Week 2		**4.** Abs and strength training, 30 minutes	**5.** Interval training				**6.** Uphill jog, 15 minutes
Week 3			**7.** Aerobic conditioning, 20 minutes				**8.** Abs and strength training
Week 4					**9.** Stretching, swimming for 30 minutes	**10.** Interval training	
Week 1							
Week 2	**11.** Abs and strength training, 60 minutes	**12.** Interval training on track					**13.** Cross-training, 30 minutes
Week 3							
Week 4							
Week 1	**14.** Belly burners and tire swings	**15.** Spinning class, 45 minutes				**16.** Belly burners and strength training, 60 minutes	

Week 2							
Week 3	**17.** Calf raises and breadbasket weaving						
Week 4			**18.** Jog for 60 minutes		**19.** Interval training	**20.** Strength squats and neck raises, 50 minutes	

Now, calorie-wise this is much better, of course—and you can add that up to be complete. Using our arbitrary 300 average, you burned 6,000 calories. Twice as much. But the real value is that if you do it this way, and you get to workout 20, you are building that bridge (figure 8). Now you will be at the catching point because of the transformation that occurred in between the workouts when you finished the list. This is a critical point. Following a quit and restart, the in-between time is blank, worthless. Finishing the list and adhering to the no restart principle creates value for your in-between days, and that is what has been missing all along! *That is what will allow you, during the next three months, to feel differently—to escape from the struggle!* These otherwise hidden days are highlighted in our new table. By following only this principle of the catching point, you have unlocked these days and burned twice as many calories. Read on, my friend, read on.

	Sunday	**Monday**	**Tuesday**	**Wednesday**	**Thursday**	**Friday**	**Saturday**
Week 1	**1.** Low-impact stretching, 20 minutes	**2.** Jog for 15 minutes	**3.** Cross-training, 10 minutes	Rest			
Week 2		**4.** Abs and strength training, 30 minutes	**5.** Interval training				**6.** Uphill jog, 15 minutes
Week 3			**7.** Aerobic conditioning, 20 minutes				**8.** Abs and strength training
Week 4					**9.** Stretching, swimming for 30 minutes	**10.** Interval training	
Week 1							
Week 2	**11.** Abs and strength training, 60 minutes	**12.** Interval training on track					**13.** Cross-training, 30 minutes
Week 3							
Week 4							

Week 1	**14.** Belly burners and tire swings	**15.** Spinning class, 45 minutes				**16.** Belly burners and strength training, 60 minutes	
Week 2							
Week 3	**17.** Calf raises and breadbasket weaving						
Week 4			**18.** Jog for 60 minutes		**19.** Interval training	**20.** Strength squats and neck raises, 50 minutes	

Erasing Time

Since we're discussing disruption of the space-time continuum, one other principle that belongs in this chapter is the idea of erasing time. When you wake up on a morning of traditional calorie restriction, you have what seems like 10,000 hours to go until bedtime. The reason for this is that every minute a dieter is abstaining from food that they want seems to stretch out to infinity. It becomes unbearable. That said, every minute spent working out, planning workouts, researching programs, buying exercise clothes, chatting in chat rooms about working out, and so on accomplishes the opposite! Not only are you not likely to consume large amounts of unwanted calories (I say unwanted because these are the "habit" meals or "emotional eating" episodes that don't really help you with recovery), but time passes. Instead of those minutes stretching out to infinity making abstinence essentially impossible, they are passed through to the langoliers, and you are on your way that much quicker.

CHAPTER 8—

Train Smart

Whoever said to fight fire with fire better rethink that, because all I've got now in my kitchen is more fire.

— Anonymous

Training is a calculated strike. A planned stressor. You do it to initiate adaptation.

— Matt Linnevers, strength and conditioning coach

THE ABSOLUTE SOLE PURPOSE of exercise is to stimulate recovery and change. It has no inherent value and accomplishes nothing else. Thinking that you have the capacity to lose weight through exercise is like saying you are going to empty a pool with a red Solo cup. Just as the cup is too small to ever make any significant change in the size of the pool, so is the average exercise capacity too small to ever impact weight loss. You should view and use exercise as a way to change your body's structure so that in the long run your metabolism is altered, your thinking is different, and your lifestyle is changed.

Thinking that you have the capacity to lose weight through exercise is like saying you are going to empty a pool with a red Solo cup.

Our first priority, before we start feverishly trying to empty the pool, is to get some different tools! Let's at least get a bucket, and at best an automatic reverse-pressure pipe system to empty the pool, right?

You've seen to this point how to create space in your program, and how critical the recovery and rewiring that takes place during these days actually is. In this chapter we discuss how to ultimately manage these days, and when you will do what. Your global plan is aimed to induce and support change on your off days.

This or That

An instructor of mine teaches a complex martial art in terms of "this" or "that." He realized that because there was so much to know, lessons would often get jumbled up in the students' heads and we would be frozen with indecision. He simplified it by grouping everything into this, or that. The true brilliance in this teaching strategy, though, was not that he simply made two lists so things would be easier to remember but that he taught them in symbiotic pairs that were inversely related.[8]

For example, imagine sumo wrestlers. The goal in a sumo wrestling match is to somehow get your opponent outside a drawn circle. My instructor would approach this situation by simplifying the problem into this or that as push or pull. He would explain that of all the potential things one could do to get the opponent out of the circle, the problem could be reduced to pushing or pulling. That is, try pushing—if that doesn't work, pull. The advantages are (1) you can't push and pull at the same time so you aren't likely to get confused, (2) the opponent can't defend pushing and pulling at the same time, and (3) most maneuvers can be put in one or the other of those categories. Big deal, right?

> We are either actively engaged in exercise, or we are recovering and rewiring.... There aren't 5,000 principles to remember about simple carbs, complex carbs, resistance exercise, slow-twitching muscle fibers, etc. It's either this. Or that. And most importantly, the more energy we put into this, the more value we get from that.

8 OK, OK, OK, that sounded a little fancy. But seriously, read on.

Maybe to this point, but what he realized was that the harder one's opponent defended himself from being pushed out of the circle, the more he was susceptible to the pull. One actually set up the other such that it wasn't a random this or that, it was an interdependent relationship that the laws of physics would always balance out. So the more you worked to do *this*, the more likely *that* was going to happen when you switched gears—and so on until you pushed Kanji-san out of the circle. This situation can be likened to a slingshot. The farther you pull, the more potential energy you build up in the opposite direction until you let go.

This (no pun intended) is the same thing. On your way to the catching point, you are either doing this or that. You are either actively engaged in exercise, or you are recovering and rewiring. That (sorry) is it. There aren't 5,000 principles to remember about simple carbs, complex carbs, resistance exercise, slow-twitching muscle fibers, and so on. It's either this. Or that. And most importantly, the more energy you put into this, the more value you get from that. The more time you spend resting, sleeping, reducing stress, and eating, the more force you will have when you switch gears back to the workout, and vice versa. The more you manage to put into the workout, the more your body will change and adapt in response, and so on.

Just as my instructor provided over time many potential maneuvers of the pull or push variety to select from, so shall this book provide you with several different options to choose from on a given day that fall into either the exercise or rest and recovery buckets. The order in which you pick from these buckets, as according to your own body, schedule, external stressors, etc., will then determine the pattern of your 84 days. So far, we've only included "extra days" and shaded them as in the last table. These would fall into the rest and recovery bucket. We could shade the exercise days differently and give a sample pattern, as below.

	Sunday	Monday	Tuesday	Wednesday	Thursday	Friday	Saturday
Week 1	**1.** Low-impact stretching, 20 minutes	**2.** Jog for 15 minutes	**3.** Cross-training, 10 minutes	Rest			
Week 2		**4.** Abs and strength training, 30 minutes	**5.** Interval training				**6.** Uphill jog, 15 minutes

Week 3			**7.** Aerobic conditioning, 20 minutes				**8.** Abs and strength training
Week 4					**9.** Stretching, swimming for 30 minutes	**10.** Interval training	
Week 1							
Week 2	**11.** Abs and strength training, 60 minutes	**12.** Interval training on track					**13.** Cross training, 30 minutes
Week 3							
Week 4							
Week 1	**14.** Belly burners and tire swings	**15.** Spinning class, 45 minutes				**16.** Belly burners and strength training, 60 minutes	
Week 2							
Week 3	**17.** Calf raises and breadbasket weaving						
Week 4			**18.** Jog for 60 minutes		**19.** Interval training	**20.** Strength squats and neck raises, 50 minutes	

The person who followed this schedule would have gotten to the catching point and would be ready to succeed in his or her traditional exercise program of choice, assuming they tuned in to their body's signals and balanced this and that.

Introducing the Workouts

The workouts themselves are designed with a two-pronged goal in mind. First, induce adaptation and change in the body during the off days, and second—to progress. *The adaptation we want is a reorganization of our molecular structures that will lead to increased exercise capacity.* Now, this sentence is sort of buried here in chapter 8, but it really represents the essence of the entire book. Said another way, *at the catching point, your body will have adapted to perform increased work through exercise*, and you will be able to do what successful people are doing with regard to exercise—you will have an effective system for emptying that pool.

The workouts are positioned with absolute intention. That is, every movement and every combination has been precisely selected to impose a specific demand that will lead to desired adaptation. That also sounds a bit high tech, but the concept is simple. Your body will only change in small increments (during recovery). When it is forced to change, to adapt, in small increments, it is a master adapter. The stimulus or stressor that you apply has to be relevant to the change you want. We have spent countless hours designing the program to "flip" you. To get you to the catching point, then beyond.

The specific stressor-adaptation model clears much of the smoke and mirrors. New stimulus equals new adaptation. Same stimulus equals no adaptation. Removal of stimulus equals your body tumbling back to its comfy zone of maximum efficiency (bad for body composition).

So here are a few things to know with regard to the workouts that might get your attention when you start the program.

1. There are three levels. Incremental adaptation to an incremental stimulus. Progress, or stay the same.

2. There is an intentional omission of "crunching" or "crunching and twisting" in the exercises. The function of your core is to prevent being pulled out of posture from an imposed force. When you execute these exercises properly by maintaining proper posture and a braced belly, you are doing just that. Your core is the trunk of the tree, your arms and legs are the branches. The branches should move without bending the trunk during all of the catching point workouts, thereby rendering them all core workouts. Be a tree.

3. Bang for the buck, risk vs. reward…whatever you call it, this filter has been used to select all our exercise choices and workout plans. You have limited time and limited physical resources. You'll get the most out of every workout by using exercises that produce the biggest return. You'll also use exercises that give the most benefit with the smallest risk of injury. We want you to stay healthy and be in it for the long haul.

4. There is no running. For this, we don't want you to run to get in shape; rather, you will get in shape to run later.[9]

5. All our workouts will be total-body workouts and encompass pattern-based training. We will use as many muscles as possible, in balance, to ensure the most efficient results. All the movements fall into these categories: push, pull, hip dominant, knee dominant, and core. There are countless ways to work out these patterns and plenty of progressions and regressions. Trust me that they are in there. The only issue we have is the lack of pulling in level 1 due to logistics of the home workout with no equipment. We know it, though, and will address it heavily in levels 2 and 3. More on this later.

6. There are outside-the-home workouts, including classes and the gym. The gym workouts are not necessarily harder, or easier, for that matter. The gym does, however, give you more options for progressive resistance and provides the tools you will need to progress from level 2 to level 3. You may notice omission of some popular gym equipment. This is no mistake. Don't be seduced by what others are doing. Follow the plan. There is a reason for everything.

7. You have to look up the exercises to learn how to do them properly. I tried to sort of hide this because I know some of you are going to be pissed about it at first. I don't worry too much about this, though, because you will thank me in the end. If you do not know what burpees are, read about it. Or watch an online video. Learn it on your own. Google it, as they say. Why? We are creating a new you that can independently operate and enjoy this new lifestyle. Part of that is education. Part of it is erasing time (see chapter 7). Make this your project. Trust me.

---

9 Running is awesome, but in the context of transformation you risk beating up your joints, stunting development of your efficient muscle fuel-burning model, and suffering overuse injuries, especially with a deconditioned body (many a fitness program has been ended by a stress fracture in a new runner who wasn't ready).

The Workouts

Introduction by Matt Linnevers

First, let me congratulate you on making the decision to take part in the unlocked mystery of success that has been so elusive for so long for so many. The catching point insight to the struggle is uniquely perceptive and instructive for all those who have failed to achieve their ideal body. The principles in this book have been validated time and time again during my years of experience with clients. Finding momentum is the Holy Grail. Those who find it ride it forward, never to fall back again behind that transformative point. Dr. Prologo has provided a scientific explanation for this phenomenon—and shown you the way through it.

Now you have reached the point of action. And here is the final and most important piece of advice: Enjoy the journey. Find pleasure in the process. Focus on the path. If you have to, fight your way to the catching point, because along the way there will be satisfaction, a sense of well-being, and feelings of accomplishment and control—all of which you will need for the long haul. It feels good to be the master of your body. It's all there for you at the catching point, I believe. Once you are there, you won't go back. After all, that's what this is *all* about.

Level 1: Building the First Block

This beginning level is your new introduction to intelligent exercise, and it is designed to prepare your body for tougher workouts as you progress. These beginning workouts encompass fitness concepts that embody good posture, cardio fitness, movement quality, mobility, and introduction to strength. This will be the case as you move through all the levels and expand upon what you do. You will burn those pesky carbohydrates and firm up the flabby parts while your body learns. This also starts the road to bulletproofing those joints and becoming injury resistant.

The exercises prescribed here all have a specific purpose, as mentioned earlier. So no skipping, and always be mindful of your form. Correct form is super important. More important than number of reps. Always remember that exercises are a tool to meet an end, they are not the end themselves. You want to maximize the effect by performing them properly, not give yourself gold stars for completing an ineffective workout. You want to build a solid foundation for your fitness future.

The workouts of level 1 are designed to be done in "circuit" fashion, in sequence right down the list, then repeat. The goal is to get to the point where you can do as much of the workout with as little rest as possible. Don't push too hard in the beginning. First try to get through two exercises in a row, then three, and on up. If you can get through all of the exercises in a row without stopping, take a rest before you begin the series again. You should also work to repeat the series three times. Rest as needed between sequences. Begin to build walls behind you, slowly but surely, step by step. Begin to transform.

What you will need:[10]

1. A pair of tennis, cross-training, or running shoes.

2. A small indoor area (winter) or a small outdoor area (summer).

3. A sidewalk to walk down safely.

4. Comfortable clothing that moves freely with your body.

5. A water bottle to stay refreshed.

6. Yellow, green, and blue mini bands from the sporting goods store. (The colors designate the level of resistance they provide.)

7. A chair and a stair.

8. A timer (cell phone, stopwatch, egg timer, etc.).

10 We tried to keep this stuff to a minimum, but remember—we aren't trying to sell gimmicks, we are trying to change people. And we need some stuff to do that. ☺

Level 1 Walk	
BRISK WALK	**To be done 1 time through**

It is important early on to get moving. The key here is to walk at a brisk pace, arms moving (rather than a "stroll"). Elevate your heart rate a bit and breathe some air. Outside is better, even if it's snowy, raining, hot, cold, etc. Walk in the park, down the street—anywhere. Soak up some fresh air and enjoy your surroundings. If you have a dog, take him or her along; they probably need it as well. Start at 20 minutes and increase by 10-minute increments according to how you feel.

Burpee Challenge

The burpee challenge is an internal challenge against your own progress. Try to get as many burpees in one day—anytime during the day—as you can. Two here, 10 there, etc. The more the better. Try to beat your previous score.

>15

>25

>35

>50

Level 1 Alpha		
WARM-UP	**To be done 1 time through**	
	Exercises	**Time/Repetitions**
	Upper Body Lat/Shoulder Stretch	30 seconds
	Standing Hamstring/ Groin Stretch	30 seconds
	Standing Calf Stretch	30 seconds
	Half-Kneeling Quad Stretch	30 seconds
	Seated T-spine Mobilizer	30 seconds
	Supine Glute Stretch	30 seconds
WORKOUT	**To be done 3 times through**	
	Exercises	**Time/Repetitions**
	Butt Kicks	30 seconds
	Inchworms	10
	Glute Bridges	12
	Mini Band Walks	20
	High Knees Marching	30 seconds
	Elevated Plank Hold	30 seconds
	Side-to-Side Lunges	20

Level 1 Beta		
WARM-UP	**To be done 1 time through**	
	Exercises	**Time/Repetitions**
	Upper Body Lat/Shoulder Stretch	30 seconds
	Standing Hamstring/Groin Stretch	30 seconds
	Standing Calf Stretch	30 seconds
	Half-Kneeling Quad Stretch	30 seconds
	Seated T-spine Mobilizer	30 seconds
	Supine Glute Stretch	30 seconds
WORKOUT	**To be done 3 times through**	
	Exercises	**Time/Repetitions**
	Prisoner Squats	12
	Mountain Climbers	40
	Side Plank	30 seconds
	Punch and Bob	60 seconds
	Birddogs	12
	Mini Band Walks	20
	Elevated Push-Ups	12
	Sideways Shuffle Touch	20

Level 1 Gamma		
WARM-UP	**To be done 1 time through**	
	Exercises	**Time/Repetitions**
	Upper Body Lat/Shoulder Stretch	30 seconds
	Standing Hamstring/Groin Stretch	30 seconds
	Standing Calf Stretch	30 seconds
	Half-Kneeling Quad Stretch	30 seconds
	Seated T-spine Mobilizer	30 seconds
	Supine Glute Stretch	30 seconds
WORKOUT	**To be done 3 times through**	
	Exercises	**Time/Repetitions**
	Step Up Alternating	20
	Elevated Plank Hold	30 seconds
	Inchworms	10
	Split Squats	12
	Leg Swings	12
	Donkey Kicks	20
	Half Jacks	20
	Chair Dips	10

Level 1 Delta		
WARM-UP	**To be done 1 time through**	
	Exercises	**Time/Repetitions**
	Upper Body Lat/Shoulder Stretch	30 seconds
	Standing Hamstring/ Groin Stretch	30 seconds
	Standing Calf Stretch	30 seconds
	Half-Kneeling Quad Stretch	30 seconds
	Seated T-spine Mobilizer	30 seconds
	Supine Glute Stretch	30 seconds
WORKOUT	**To be done 3 times through**	
	Exercises	**Time/Repetitions**
	Step Lunges with Reach	20
	Butt Kicks	30 seconds
	Elevated Close-Grip Push-Ups	12
	Punch/Punch/Side Kick	30 seconds
	Wall Scap Retractions	12
	Wall Push Runner Core	12
	Invisible Jump Rope	12

Level 1 Epsilon		
WARM-UP	**To be done 1 time through**	
	Exercises	**Time/Repetitions**
	Upper Body Lat/Shoulder Stretch	30 seconds
	Standing Hamstring/Groin Stretch	30 seconds
	Standing Calf Stretch	30 seconds
	Half-Kneeling Quad Stretch	30 seconds
	Seated T-spine Mobilizer	30 seconds
	Supine Glute Stretch	30 seconds
WORKOUT	**To be done 3 times through**	
	Exercises	**Time/Repetitions**
	Single-Leg Dead Lifts	20
	No Moneys	12
	Mini Band Walks	20
	Wall-Sit Arm Circles	45 seconds
	Elevated Plank Hold	30 seconds
	Picking Up Change	30 seconds
	Single-Leg Squats	20

Level 1 Zeta		
WARM-UP	**To be done 1 time through**	
	Exercises	**Time/Repetitions**
	Upper Body Lat/Shoulder Stretch	30 seconds
	Standing Hamstring/ Groin Stretch	30 seconds
	Standing Calf Stretch	30 seconds
	Half-Kneeling Quad Stretch	30 seconds
	Seated T-spine Mobilizer	30 seconds
	Supine Glute Stretch	30 seconds
WORKOUT	**To be done 3 times through**	
	Exercises	**Time/Repetitions**
	Single-Leg Glute Bridges	12
	Spider Man Mountain Climber	30 seconds
	Step Lunges/Sideways Lunges with Reach	20
	Bird Dogs	12
	High Knee March/Fast Feet	10–15 seconds, 3 times
	Wall Scap Retractions	12
	Side Plank Hold	30 seconds per side

Level 1 Eta		
WARM-UP	**To be done 1 time through**	
	Exercises	**Time/Repetitions**
	Upper Body Lat/Shoulder Stretch	30 seconds
	Standing Hamstring/Groin Stretch	30 seconds
	Standing Calf Stretch	30 seconds
	Half-Kneeling Quad Stretch	30 seconds
	Seated T-spine Mobilizer	30 seconds
	Supine Glute Stretch	30 seconds
WORKOUT	**To be done 3 times through**	
	Exercises	**Time/Repetitions**
	45-Degree Lunges	20
	Elevated Push-Ups	12
	Glute Bridges	12
	Sideways Walking Planks	30 seconds
	Sideways Shuffle Touches	30 seconds
	Punch/Punch/Knee	30 seconds
	Squat to Stand with Mini Band	10

Level 1 Theta		
WARM-UP	**To be done 1 time through**	
	Exercises	**Time/Repetitions**
	Upper Body Lat/Shoulder Stretch	30 seconds
	Standing Hamstring/Groin Stretch	30 seconds
	Standing Calf Stretch	30 seconds
	Half-Kneeling Quad Stretch	30 seconds
	Seated T-spine Mobilizer	30 seconds
	Supine Glute Stretch	30 seconds
WORKOUT	**To be done 3 times through**	
	Exercises	**Time/Repetitions**
	Mini Band Walks	20
	Glute Bridges	12
	Sideways Walking Planks	30 seconds
	Mountain Climbers	30 seconds
	Sideways Shuffle Touches	30 seconds
	Wall-Sit Arm Circles	45 seconds
	Front Kick/Front Kick/ Punch/Punch	30 seconds

Level 1 Iota		
WARM-UP	**To be done 1 time through**	
	Exercises	**Time/Repetitions**
	Upper Body Lat/Shoulder Stretch	30 seconds
	Standing Hamstring/Groin Stretch	30 seconds
	Standing Calf Stretch	30 seconds
	Half-Kneeling Quad Stretch	30 seconds
	Seated T-spine Mobilizer	30 seconds
	Supine Glute Stretch	30 seconds
WORKOUT	**To be done 3 times through**	
	Exercises	**Time/Repetitions**
	Elevated Push-Ups	12
	Picking Up Change	30 seconds
	Glute Bridges	12
	Step Lunges/Sideways Lunges with Reach	20
	Elevated Plank Holds	30
	Inchworms	10
	No Moneys	12

Level 2: The Transition Begins

Perform these exercises in circuit fashion, in sequence, one after the other with minimal rest, just like before. Remember: technique, technique, technique. This is most important. Also, we will take advantage of the treadmill, stationary bike, and stair climber for workout finishers.

What you will need:

1. A Swiss ball.
2. Resistance bands with handles (for rowing).
3. A timer (cell phone, stopwatch, egg timer, etc.).
4. Access to a gym or rec center.[11]

LEVEL 2 WARM-UP[12]

A. Butt Kicks: 15 seconds

B. High Knees: 15 seconds

C. Lateral Shuffle Touches: 15 seconds

D. Step Lunges with Reach: 8 per side

E. Lateral Lunges: 8 per side

F. Straight-Leg Swings: 8 per side

G. Inchworms: 8

H. Mini Band Walks: 10 per side

I. Glute Bridges: 10

J. Wall Scap Retractions: 15

K. Swiss Ball Shoulder/Lat Stretch: 8 per side

L. Swiss Ball Pec/Shoulder Stretch: 20 seconds per side

Level 2 Walk	
BRISK WALK	**To be done 1 time through**
No warm-up needed. This walk needs to be a bit faster paced and longer than the level 1 walk. Hills or, if available, stairs would be great additions if available. Walk for 45 minutes.	

11 This one is optional. See text regarding the value of getting out, but if it is a barrier to continuing, exchange it for a home option.

12 *Never* skip this warmup, please. It is probably the most critical element of your progression and is crucial for development of mobility and functionality and for injury prevention.

Level 2 Alpha		
WARM-UP	**To be done 1 time through**	
	Exercises	**Time/Repetitions**
	Butt Kicks	15 seconds
	High Knees	15 seconds
	Lateral Shuffle Touches	15 seconds
	Step Lunges with Reach	8 per side
	Lateral Lunges	8 per side
	Straight-Leg Swings	8 per side
	Inchworms	8
	Mini Band Walks	10 per side
	Glute Bridges	10
	Wall Scap Retractions	15
	Swiss Ball Shoulder/Lat Stretch	8 per side
	Swiss Ball Pec/Shoulder Stretch	20 seconds per side
WORKOUT	**To be done 3 times through**	
	Exercises	**Time/Repetitions**
	Single-Leg Glute Bridge with Mini Band	10 per side
	Tube Rows	15
	Swiss Ball Ham Curl/Hip Extension	12
	Tube Split Squat/Over-head Press	10 per side
	Swiss Ball Plank with Circles	30 seconds
	Tube Bicep Curls	15
	Swiss Ball Push-Ups	15

Level 2 Beta		
WARM-UP	**To be done 1 time through**	
	Exercises	**Time/Repetitions**
	Butt Kicks	15 seconds
	High Knees	15 seconds
	Lateral Shuffle Touches	15 seconds
	Step Lunges with Reach	8 per side
	Lateral Lunges	8 per side
	Straight-Leg Swings	8 per side
	Inchworms	8
	Mini Band Walks	10 per side
	Glute Bridges	10
	Wall Scap Retractions	15
	Swiss Ball Shoulder/Lat Stretch	8 per side
	Swiss Ball Pec/Shoulder Stretch	20 seconds per
WORKOUT	**To be done 3 times through**	
	Exercises	**Time/Repetitions**
	Squat Jumps	10
	Tube Rows	15
	Single-Leg Deadlift	10 per side
	Tube Lat Raises	12
	Swiss Ball Push-Ups	12
	Reverse Lunges	12 per side
	Swiss Ball Plank with Circles	30 seconds

Level 2 Gamma		
WARM-UP	**To be done 1 time through**	
	Exercises	**Time/Repetitions**
	Butt Kicks	15 seconds
	High Knees	15 seconds
	Lateral Shuffle Touches	15 seconds
	Step Lunges with Reach	8 per side
	Lateral Lunges	8 per side
	Straight-Leg Swings	8 per side
	Inchworms	8
	Mini Band Walks	10 per side
	Glute Bridges	10
	Wall Scap Retractions	15
	Swiss Ball Shoulder/Lat Stretch	8 per side
	Swiss Ball Pec/Shoulder Stretch	20 seconds per
WORKOUT	**To be done 3 times through**	
	Exercises	**Time/Repetitions**
	Swiss Ball Mountain Climbers	45 seconds
	Tube Rows	15
	Tube Chop Lifts	10 per side
	Ice Skaters	45 seconds
	Push-Ups	As many as possible
	Swiss Ball Ham Curl/Hip Extensions	12
	Jump Split Squats	16

Level 2 Delta		
WARM-UP	**To be done 1 time through**	
	Exercises	**Time/Repetitions**
	Butt Kicks	15 seconds
	High Knees	15 seconds
	Lateral Shuffle Touches	15 seconds
	Step Lunges with Reach	8 per side
	Lateral Lunges	8 per side
	Straight-Leg Swings	8 per sides
	Inchworms	8
	Mini Band Walks	10 per side
	Glute Bridges	10
	Wall Scap Retractions	15
	Swiss Ball Shoulder/Lat Stretch	8 per side
	Swiss Ball Pec/Shoulder Stretch	20 seconds per side
WORKOUT	**To be done 3 times through**	
	Exercises	**Time/Repetitions**
	Single-Leg Glute Bridge with Mini Band	12 per side
	Tube Rows	15
	Burpees	10
	Sideways Lunges	12 per side
	Rear Foot Elevated Split Squat	12 per side
	Tube Lateral Raises/Front Raises	12
	Swiss Ball Plank with Circles	30 seconds

Level 2 Epsilon (Gym)		
WARM-UP	**To be done 1 time through**	
	Exercises	**Time/Repetitions**
	Butt Kicks	15 seconds
	High Knees	15 seconds
	Lateral Shuffle Touches	15 seconds
	Step Lunges with Reach	8 per
	Lateral Lunges	8 per
	Straight-Leg Swings	8 per
	Inchworms	8
	Mini Band Walks	10 per
	Glute Bridges	10
	Wall Scap Retractions	15
	Swiss Ball Shoulder/Lat Stretch	8 per side
	Swiss Ball Pec/Shoulder Stretch	20 seconds per
WORKOUT	**To be done 3 times through**	
	Exercises	**Time/Repetitions**
	Dumbbell 3-Point Row	12 per side
	Goblet Squats	12
	Swiss Ball Dumbbell Press	12
	Kettle Bell Swings	12
	Half-Kneeling Overhead Press	12 per side
	Band-Assisted Chin-Up	10
	Swiss Ball Plank with Circles	45 seconds
	FINISHER: Stair climber or Incline Treadmill Walk	15 minutes

Level 2 Zeta (Gym)		
WARM-UP	To be done 1 time through	
	Exercises	Time/Repetitions
	Butt Kicks	15 seconds
	High Knees	15 seconds
	Lateral Shuffle Touches	15 seconds
	Step Lunges with Reach	8 per side
	Lateral Lunges	8 per side
	Straight-Leg Swings	8 per side
	Inchworms	8
	Mini Band Walks	10 per side
	Glute Bridges	10
	Wall Scap Retractions	15
	Swiss Ball Shoulder/Lat Stretch	8 per side
	Swiss Ball Pec/Shoulder Stretch	20 seconds per
WORKOUT	To be done 3 times through	
	Exercises	Time/Repetitions
	TRX Row—Standing	12
	TRX Single-Leg Squats	12 per side
	TRX Fly Press	12
	TRX Ham Curl/Bridges	12
	TRX Runner Plank	10 per side
	TRX Face Pull/Extension Rotation	12
	TRX Sprint Start	10 per side
	FINISHER: Bike, medium pace	15 minutes
WARM-UP	To be done 1 time through	

	Exercises	Time/Repetitions
	Butt Kicks	15 seconds
	High Knees	15 seconds
	Lateral Shuffle Touches	15 seconds
	Step Lunges with Reach	8 per side
	Lateral Lunges	8 per side
	Straight-Leg Swings	8 per side
	Inchworms	8
	Mini Band Walks	10 per side
	Glute Bridges	10
	Wall Scap Retractions	15
	Swiss Ball Shoulder/Lat Stretch	8 per side
	Swiss Ball Pec/Shoulder Stretch	20 seconds per side
WORKOUT	**To be done 3 times through**	
	Exercises	**Time/Repetitions**
	Dumbbell Bench Single-Leg Glute Bridges	10 per side
	Dumbbell 3-Point Row	12 per side
	Dumbbell Step Lunges	12 per side
	Bench Push-Ups	Max
	Goblet Squats	12
	Feet-Elevated Side Plank	30 seconds per side
	Dumbbell Bicep Curls	12
	FINISHER: Stair Climber or Incline Treadmill Walk	15 minutes

Level 2 Theta (Gym)		
WARM-UP	**To be done 1 time through**	
	Exercises	**Time/Repetitions**
	Butt Kicks	15 seconds
	High Knees	15 seconds
	Lateral Shuffle Touches	15 seconds
	Step Lunges with Reach	8 per side
	Lateral Lunges	8 per side
	Straight-Leg Swings	8 per side
	Inchworms	8
	Mini Band Walks	10 per side
	Glute Bridges	10
	Wall Scap Retractions	15
	Swiss Ball Shoulder/Lat Stretch	8 per side
	Swiss Ball Pec/Shoulder Stretch	20 seconds per side
WORKOUT	**To be done 3 times through**	
	Exercises	**Time/Repetitions**
	Kettle Bell Swing	12
	Lat Pull-Downs	12
	Rear Foot Elevated Split Squat Dumbbell	10 per side
	Swiss Ball Alternating Press	10 per side
	Dumbbell Single-Leg Dead Lifts	10 per side
	Front to Side to Side Plank	30 seconds per side
	Barbell Row	12
	FINISHER: Bike, medium pace	15 minutes

Level 2 Iota (Gym)		
WARM-UP	**To be done 1 time through**	
	Exercises	**Time/Repetitions**
	Butt Kicks	15 seconds
	High Knees	15 seconds
	Lateral Shuffle Touches	15 seconds
	Step Lunges with Reach	8 per side
	Lateral Lunges	8 per side
	Straight-Leg Swings	8 per side
	Inchworms	8
	Mini Band Walks	10 per side
	Glute Bridges	10
	Wall Scap Retractions	15
	Swiss Ball Shoulder/Lat Stretch	8 per side
	Swiss Ball Pec/Shoulder Stretch	20 seconds per side
WORKOUT	**To be done 3 times through**	
	Exercises	**Time/Repetitions**
	TRX Row, Standing	12
	Bench Press Push-Up	Max
	Dumbbell Reverse Lunges	12 per side
	Band-Assisted Chin Ups	12
	Dumbbell Step-Ups	12 per side
	Dumbbell Bicep CurlsW	12 per side
	FINISHER: Stair Climber or Incline Treadmill Walk	15 minutes

Level 3: Metamorphosis

If you've made it here you have accomplished quite a bit by now. Level 3 is a bit different, in keeping with your ongoing change. Embrace your newfound strength. Be gratified that you are taking control of your ship. Get addicted to the feeling. Almost there.

Level 3 Alpha		
WARM-UP	**To be done 1 time through**	
	Exercises	**Time/Repetitions**
	Butt Kicks	15 seconds
	High Knees	15 seconds
	Lateral Shuffle Touches	15 seconds
	Step Lunges with Reach	8 per side
	Lateral Lunges	8 per side
	Straight-Leg Swings	8 per side
	Inchworms	8
	Mini Band Walks	10 per side
	Glute Bridges	10
	Wall Scap Retractions	15
	Swiss Ball Shoulder/Lat Stretch	8 per side
	Swiss Ball Pec/Shoulder Stretch	20 seconds per side
WORKOUT	**To be done 3 times through**	
	Exercises	**Time/Repetitions**
	Prisoner Squats	15
	Burpees	10
	Jump Split Squats	10 per side
	Mountain Climbers	45 seconds
	Push-Up/Sideways Move/Push-Up	45 seconds
	Dying Bugs	45 seconds

	Tube Row/Face Pull	12/10
WARM-UP	**To be done 1 time through**	
	Exercises	**Time/Repetitions**
	Butt Kicks	15 seconds
	High Knees	15 seconds
	Lateral Shuffle Touches	15 seconds
	Step Lunges with Reach	8 per side
	Lateral Lunges	8 per side
	Straight-Leg Swings	8 per side
	Inchworms	8
	Mini Band Walks	10 per side
	Glute Bridges	10
	Wall Scap Retractions	15
	Swiss Ball Shoulder/Lat Stretch	8 per side
	Swiss Ball Pec/Shoulder Stretch	20 sec per side
WORKOUT	**To be done 3 times through**	
	Exercises	**Time/Repetitions**
	Sideways Shuffle Touches	45 seconds
	Lunge Matrix	8 per side
	Tube Palloff Press	12 per side
	Tube Row/Face Pull	12/10
	Super Slow Push-Up	Max
	Picking Up Change	30 seconds
	Feet-Elevated Side Plank	45 seconds/per side
WARM-UP	**To be done 1 time through**	
	Exercises	**Time/Repetitions**
	Butt Kicks	15 seconds

	High Knees	15 seconds
	Lateral Shuffle Touches	15 seconds
	Step Lunges with Reach	8 per side
	Lateral Lunges	8 per side
	Straight-Leg Swings	8 per side
	Inchworms	8
	Mini Band Walks	10 per side
	Glute Bridges	10
	Wall Scap Retractions	15
	Swiss Ball Shoulder/Lat Stretch	8 per side
	Swiss Ball Pec/Shoulder Stretch	20 seconds per side
WORKOUT	**To be done 3 times through**	
	Exercises	**Time/Repetitions**
	Jump Squats	15
	Tube Lateral Raise/ Front Raise	12/10
	Dying Bugs	45 seconds
	Ice Skaters	45 seconds
	Tube Row/Face Pull	12/10
	Tube Split Squat/Over-head Press	12 per side
	Swiss Ball Ham Curl/ Hip Extension	15
WARM-UP	**To be done 1 time through**	
	Exercises	**Time/Repetitions**
	Butt Kicks	15 seconds
	High Knees	15 seconds
	Lateral Shuffle Touches	15 seconds
	Step Lunges with Reach	8 per side

	Lateral Lunges	8 per side
	Straight-Leg Swings	8 per side
	Inchworms	8
	Mini Band Walks	10 per side
	Glute Bridges	10
	Wall Scap Retractions	15
	Swiss Ball Shoulder/Lat Stretch	8 per side
	Swiss Ball Pec/Shoulder Stretch	20 sec per side
WORKOUT	**To be done 3 times through**	
	Exercises	**Time/Repetitions**
	Spider Man Mountain Climbers with Push-Up	45 seconds
	Swiss Ball Plank with Circles	45 seconds
	Sideways Shuffle Touches	45 seconds
	Tube Row/Face Pull	12/10
	Fast Feet/Jump Knee Tucks	45 seconds
	Tube Palloff Press	12 per side
	Single-Leg Glute Bridge with Mini Band	12 per side
WARM-UP	**To be done 1 time through**	
	Exercises	**Time/Repetitions**
	Butt Kicks	15 seconds
	High Knees	15 seconds
	Lateral Shuffle Touches	15 seconds
	Step Lunges with Reach	8 per side
	Lateral Lunges	8 per side
	Straight-Leg Swings	8 per side
	Inchworms	8

	Mini Band Walks	10 per side
	Glute Bridges	10
	Wall Scap Retractions	15
	Swiss Ball Shoulder/Lat Stretch	8 per side
	Swiss Ball Pec/Shoulder Stretch	20 seconds per side
WORKOUT	**To be done 3 times through**	
	Exercises	**Time/Repetitions**
	Step Lunges/Tube Curl	10/12
	Swill Ball Rollout Holds	10
	Fast Feet Burpees	12
	Swill Ball Elevated-Feet Pike Walk to Overhead Push-Up	10
	Squat Jumps with Bounces	12
	Clapping Push-Ups	10
	Dying Bugs	45 seconds

At the end of the catching point program, you will enjoy a number of benefits:

1. You will be able to step into a traditional program and succeed because you will have the exercise capacity to do what you cannot do now.

2. You will have rewired your brain to crave exercise and clean foods.

3. You will be educated and independent.

4. Though I hesitate to mention this because I don't want it to be a distraction, you will have begun *really* tipping the caloric balance in your favor.[13]

This key change will result in back-feeding of messages to the brain to keep the momentum going. Eat clean, exercise more, feel great! That cycle feeds off itself, and the lifestyle "catches on." In the long run, this plan will itself tip caloric balance and so forth. What you need to do for this program is progress *to some degree* by the 84-day mark. Workout 2 is not the same as workout 1. Workout 8 is quantitatively more than workout 4.

So while we will concentrate globally on getting to the highest number workout we can during the 84 days, so shall we concentrate on getting as much done in each workout as possible. The overarching principles of the program make their way down into each workout. That is, if the directions say 10 repetitions, and you get 8—fabulous. If it isn't going perfectly or you don't feel pretty, finish anyway. A valuable tool while doing this is to concentrate on your feelings *after* the workout. If you look forward to resting at the end of the day and watching TV and snacking, think about how great that will feel when this is over. If you like to sit in hot tubs, nap, read, or play Xbox, think about how great you are going to feel doing those things after this is done. You are earning real relaxation. The workout will give you a sense of progress, accomplishment, and peace that is enjoyable. Keep those future situations in your mind during the workout.

You are earning real relaxation.

If interested in taking it a step further, imagine that your recreation time *depends* on finishing the workout. Realize that the positive feelings that come from being involved in this program and changing your life follow from the calculated stress you are applying now. Stress and adapt, stress and adapt, stress and adapt. Then revel in your change and survival.

---

13 When you start exercising, you probably burn 100 or 150 calories per workout. By the end of this program, your capacity will have increased such that your calorie burn will actually start to matter in the big picture. The truth is, distance runners don't even care about calorie intake. They burn so many calories that it doesn't matter. My guess is that to this point you haven't burned any significant amount of calories to impact the balance. At the end of the program, your efforts will be worth noting in the grand scheme of calorie balance, and the scale will start to shift in your favor (as opposed to throwing pebbles into the ocean with your 50 repeats of workout 1).

Music

Music is an incredible force for linking mind and body.[84] There is a reason 90 percent of successful people at the gym are wearing headphones.[85] The sound compilations directly affect the signals being sent out by your brain to your body. Music induces the mind-body interaction in an antegrade fashion (from brain to body vs. retrograde from body to brain as in recovery techniques such as massage). Let's face it: working out can suck. Especially if it's just going through a list of repetitive motions that have really no emotional link for you. It's much easier for a professional dancer to get through 100 leaps than it would be for us because she has a link in her brain to drive the training. She can generate those antegrade mind-body signals by picturing her upcoming performance and the standing ovation she may receive. Without that link, the average person is left with a mundane task of meaningless exercises. Music serves as that drive and link. Make a playlist, wear headphones, be inspired.

Along the same lines are social workouts. This, I realize, is potentially delicate ground for readers of this book. On the one hand, I do not want anyone to be discouraged or put a roadblock in anyone's progress. If the idea of going in public and/or trying to keep up with others puts you into a cold sweat, then forget it. Remember, goal number one is *to get stuff done*. If a social workout serves to counteract goal number one, then bypass it. Do what you have to do to get stuff done; do not allow things that give you pause or slow you down to demand your attention. That said, if you can tolerate it, there are immense benefits to working out with or around others, not dissimilar to music.[86] The presence of others can induce the same antegrade signals found with music or visualization. Moreover, it may serve as a long-term motivator through relationships and alternative rewards (see chapter 11).

One final word about the workouts. Do them and forget them. Like changing your oil. You need to get it done, but don't let the program define your life. You are just adding these things in (workouts, recovery interventions) without making grandiose changes to your life. So work out, feel good about it, then forget it. It will help you stave off burnout and diminishing returns.

Burnout and Diminishing Returns

In order to balance these days appropriately, it is important to understand the concept of burnout. Burnout is another real change in your body's chemistry that blocks your progress or induces you to quit. All of these things manifest themselves through the same neural network described above. They are actual chemical changes that result in different signals being sent to your brain, which in turn results in the brain acting responsibly and shutting you down.[87] Remember, in the end, we are all human beings with survival mechanisms in place. Our bodies have evolved over time to survive and reproduce. *Your body knows what it can handle.*

We need to back up here for one second, because the mentioning of limits and thresholds begs us to recognize the school of thought that says "push beyond your limits" and "go beyond what you thought possible." I completely agree that limits are arbitrary—however, they should be readjusted, not ignored.

For example, a baseball pitcher who really wants to play in the major leagues may practice and practice, throwing 100 balls a day. This pitcher really is in the same position as readers of this book who have a fitness goal. Both have a goal and are trying to reach said goal. If the pitcher throws and throws and throws until his shoulder starts to ache, he will likely get a bit better. At that point, though, if the pitcher ignores the signal being sent to him by his brain that his shoulder hurts and keeps throwing because his spirit is stronger than his limits (he fights fire with fire), he is likely to suffer a serious injury, or at minimum, his progress will be significantly slowed. He will begin to see less and less improvement for the same workouts, i.e., experiencing diminishing returns. Once in the zone of diminishing returns, the pitcher starts to get frustrated and tired, his mechanics break down, and he either gets hurt (as above) or just quits. Sound familiar?

Elite athletes know this well. They are precisely tuned in to the messages their brains send them about their bodies, and they respond. They understand these messages and listen to them like they are gospel, using recovery as the road to fitness improvement and overall health. They are constantly *resetting their limits*, which is what you are trying to do with this program. You aren't technically pushing through limits; you are changing your body at the molecular level so that your limits change and you can accomplish more.

Burnout and diminishing returns are negative forces that will contribute to failure. They arise when we stubbornly stick to a generic program in a blind effort to get in shape. No doubt they have contributed to a failed attempt by most readers of this book in the past. Burnout and diminishing returns only happen when you ignore your body's message that it needs time to recover, rewire, and readjust. By ignoring these messages, you stress your body when it is weak, sending alerts to the brain that your body is in danger, and—you guessed it—the brain responds by convincing you to quit in the interest of survival.[88]

Importantly, this is not voodoo or some subjective take on exercise. These are facts. Real molecules circulate in the blood that signal to the brain to shut it down. Several studies have confirmed disruptions in glucose, lactate, ammonia, glycerol, white blood cells, oxygen consumption, red blood cells, adrenaline molecules, and heart rate in humans confirmed to be into diminishing returns.[89–92] Studies have further shown that the best way to monitor these levels in order to maintain a positive recovery balance and avoid "running off the cliff" (chapter 5) is to self-report and evaluate them.[89, 91, 93, 94]

For you in the catching point program, it will be important to receive these messages and react accordingly. Specifically, when your body sends the message that it is recovering and building a wall so that you don't go backwards, you must rest and allow it to do so. You must then supplement your diet with things that nurture recovery and activities that promote rewiring and readjustment. You must not work out again! This is probably (after hunger) the most powerful force leading folks to quit their programs.

The body is recovering and trying to progress and solidify your new level. But often, because the program says to restrict food and work out, you do—and the brain shuts you down, through messages exactly like those the pitcher gets: frustration from injury and diminishing returns. The key for you and the pitcher is to rest, supplement, and contribute to your recovery for a few days, after which you will return to the workout portion of your program stronger, motivated, and with a shiny new brick wall behind you keeping you safe from a backward fall.

So how do you recognize this message? Easy, easy, easy. The very first message that your brain will send you during this brick-laying, molecule-changing recovery phase is not to exercise! Seriously. That feeling you get two or three days in that you just want to chuck the whole idea of losing weight is not because you are a quitter. It is a message from your brain to lie low while it changes your body so you can be successful. Your brain is saying, "Hang on—don't work out again just yet. I'm getting ready."

> That feeling you get two or three days in that you just want to chuck the whole idea of losing weight is not lack of willpower or your thyroid kicking in. It is a message from your brain to lie low while it changes your body so you can be successful. Your brain is saying, "Hang on—don't work out again just yet. I'm getting ready."

In the past, you interpreted this message as lack of willpower, or loss of motivation, or your thyroid kicking in. It was none of those things. Does it seem reasonable that three days after you were absolutely convinced you wanted a change in your life, wanted to diet and exercise, and lose weight, were finished with your old slob glutton ways, that you lost your motivation? In three days you had a complete change of heart? A few days prior it was important enough to buy equipment, clothes, and books and make a schedule, but now you just lost interest? Are you a schizophrenic? (Technically you would have multiple personality disorder, but let's not be picky.) No! You are the same person you were when you started, but now you are getting the message from your brain to rest and recover. Your brain is trying to help you get to the next level, but you interpret it as a loss of willpower, quit the whole thing, and go back to day 1 again in a few weeks. Ugh!

Well now you know. The very first signal your brain will send you that it is reorganizing your molecular structure is to lie low while it does so. There are some other signals as well, and they can be subtle. To help, consider figure 17 and the questionnaire in the accompanying table. If you score above 6 on the questionnaire, take a day off—and there is so much we can do to maximize these days off, so let's start adding those in.

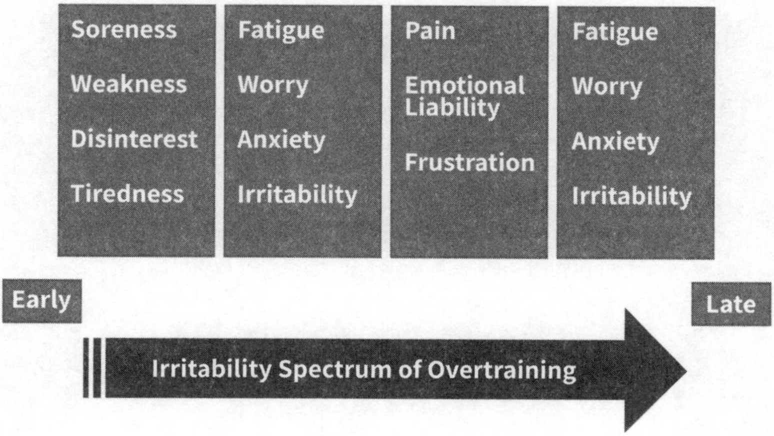

Figure 17.

Self-Assessment Questionnaire

	Yes (0 points)	Sort of (1/2 point)	No (1 point)
My home life is going well.			
Overall, I am sleeping well.			
I have been less irritable than usual.			
I think exercise is important.			
My achiness is gone.			
My injuries are better.			
I have been enjoying life.			
I have been enjoying work.			
I have been enjoying exercise.			
My temper has been good.			
My diet is improving.			
I am hopeful for the future.			
I feel strong.			
I am excited to lose some weight and get in shape.			
I don't exercise enough.			

CHAPTER 9—

The In-Between Days

The body seeks lost sleep with a vigour comparable to or greater than that displayed for food or sex.

— Jerome Siegel, Professor, Psychiatry and Biobehavioral Sciences, UCLA95

NOW WE ARE GETTING TO the epicenter of our plan. The in-between days. This is where the magic happens. On these days you must be mindful of the following variables.

Sleep

Sleep is primarily a brain thing. Thousands of articles and many books have been written on sleep as it relates to brain function, brain waves, thinking, memory, mood, and so on. The role of sleep in physical metabolic change, though, is what we care about. Simply put, sleep is the time when your body builds the scaffold. Exercise is nothing more than a stimulus for adaptation, a calculated assault on our body's muscles, lungs, heart, and nerves. Our brain then says, "Hmmph, if we are going to have to keep doing this task, I've got to change a few things." The brain, then, as the master molecular organizer, sends out messages through the extensive network described earlier to reorganize things so you can do the task. The changes the brain orders up, as mentioned in chapter 5, are called anabolic changes. These are the changes we ultimately need and must encourage. Seventy-five percent of the changes we are after will occur during sleep (the other 25 during rest). At this point in your fitness career, I would go so far as to say that adequate and extra sleep are more important than diet or exercise. Let's chew on that for a bit.

> Note that *none* of the changes to your body that are necessary to succeed occur during the workouts. The calories burned during the workouts are a drop in the bucket; they really don't matter. The purpose of the workout is to induce change that will occur during rest.

The central theme of this book and program is to reorganize your body's structure in a way that will allow you to enter the fitness world and take on traditional diet and exercise programs. Hopefully I have made the point that this reorganization occurs during rest. What exactly is happening? New molecules are being churned out for you. Like new marble for your counters or oak for your cabinets or paint for the walls in the house you are remodeling. The purpose of these molecules is to remodel *you*. Use them.

Structurally, your body is making molecules *during sleep that follows exercise* that will do the following useful things for you: strengthen your muscles; lower your blood pressure; neutralize inflammation; increase your metabolism; decrease damage caused by stress; give you energy; protect your heart; protect you from cancer; protect you from diabetes; mobilize your protective immune response so you get sick less; safeguard you from depression, injuries, and stroke; as well as make you smarter.[14, 95–111]

The hook, I am betting for my readers and friends here, is that sleeping enough will make you *eat less*. Right, eat less. Functional MRI scans of the brain have shown that people are far more interested in eating when they are sleep deprived. Moreover, sleep-deprived subjects are more driven toward unhealthy foods when given the option. Sleep-deprived subjects also have increased levels of ghrelin, the hormone that makes us feel hungry, and decreased levels of leptin, the hormone that makes us feel full. And it's not just brain MRI studies and hormone-level draws that have been done; subjects have been shown to actually eat more food and

---

14 "Stress" here is a whole host of things, from external stressors that increase cortisol levels to store fat to direct reduction (chemically and literally) of something called oxidative stress that accelerates aging.

actually gain more weight when sleep deprived, and population-based studies have shown increased BMI (body-mass index) numbers in people with less sleep hours.[110, 112–127]

Ultimately, the rest of the details underpinning those last two paragraphs get a little "sciencey," so I've put them in appendix 2—right after the riveting read about kinetic changes.

Diet

You can't build a scaffold without wood, and you can't make changes in your body's structure without the appropriate nutrients on board.[37, 128] If, while you are sleeping, your body sets out to build your scaffold so you can ultimately run a marathon, or crush the tough mudder, or go to yoga class, and there is no wood, there will be no change. The specific nutrients and foods necessary for recovery and change are as follows:

Tryptophan, Tart Cherries, Cottage Cheese, and Toast

The first three are for sleep. Although the source of tryptophan (turkey, for example) may also contribute to the scaffold, we are ultimately interested in sleeping. Tryptophan, and components of tart cherries or tart cherry juice, serve as precursors to neurotransmitters that promote sleep. That means when they are broken down as part of digestion, the pieces cross into the brain and improve sleep. Cottage cheese contains casein protein, which will slowly release overnight and keep your body from breaking down what you built to get parts for your scaffold. The toast is to fill you up, because decreased caloric intake and feeling hungry will disrupt sleep. Consider having this meal in the evening 60 minutes before going to bed.[129, 130]

Lunasin, Sweet Potato Proteins, and Polyphenols

This translates to soy, sweet potatoes, and coffee, plums, and sweet cherries. These components of your diet are key to recovery and restructuring following exercise. It is the *inclusion* of these elements to your diet that is important. Here is where we are starting to turn traditional thinking on its ear. We aren't considering these as diet replacements or the list of foods you are "allowed to eat." You *have* to add these in to your diet without consciously changing anything else. Why? Because of oxidative stress and inflammation.[131–139]

Inflammatory response is great to have in the presence of infection because it orchestrates the immune system attack on whatever bacteria or virus your kids brought home from school. It will eloquently and aggressively clear your system of the little intruder, but just like any war or retaliatory attack, it leaves damage in its wake—which is why you feel like crap when you are sick.[15] Likewise, stress on the body results in oxidative species, which are like little spikey sour balls that bounce around inside you and damage all your cells.[87, 128, 140]

> Stress on the body results in oxidative species, which are like little spikey sour balls that bounce around inside you and damage all your cells.

Just like you take vitamins and medicines when you are sick to aid your body in recovery, so shall you ingest these foods in between workouts to lessen this inflammatory response and neutralize the oxidative stress. *Remember, the goal is to keep your fire lit. Keep you feeling well and motivated and improve the status of your body. In essence make you stronger so going forward it isn't such an impossibility to tolerate these exercise programs.* So in the 48 hours following any workout, eat cherries, sweet potatoes, and soy. Drink coffee. And understand the reasoning behind these supplements is to neutralize the collateral damage that occurs during exercise and allow for rebuilding.[16]

Lysine, Glutamic Acid, and Heat Shock Proteins

A consistent theme (I hope) throughout this book has been to reduce the body's responses to exercise that make you feel like crap and zap your motivation and to accelerate and embrace the body's responses that result in rebuilding and transformation and adaptation. In keeping with this, we must now consider the heat shock proteins. These are a set of proteins that each of us has whose purpose is to respond to physical stress by adapting our bodies. These are referred to in the scientific literature as the molecular chaperones of protection and change.[25, 131, 141–143] They are your evolutionary infrastructure, meaning that they exist in the shadows,

15 Incidentally, please consider how you react when you feel sick, and you know you have an infection. You rest, you hydrate, you take vitamins and medicine, and you bide your time while your body recovers. Hmmmmm....

16 As an added bonus, these proteins have also been shown to prevent cancer and heart disease through similar mechanisms, the details of which are beyond the scope of this book. If you are interested, I would recommend starting with the referenced works.

then emerge following a stressor (like exercise) to clean up the mess and rebuild a stronger framework for next time. *These are absolutely critical to what we are trying to do through the catching point program.*

> Heat shock proteins...are referred to in the scientific literature as the molecular chaperones of protection and change.

Consider the complex engineering that is required to "earthquake-proof" a building.[144] Human beings have adapted and evolved the structure of buildings built in regions known to experience earthquakes by changing and strengthening the infrastructure of the building according to previous experienced forces. These changes are translated to reality by construction workers who actually nail together beams in this specific arrangement, rendering the building stronger and safer in the presence of a future earthquake. The body makes adjustments to its structure in the same way after being exposed to exercise—rearranging its "beams" and "nails" to a pattern more like those beyond the catching point, using heat shock proteins as its workers.

The heat shock proteins exist in two forms, or two locations in the cell depending on whether the body has been exposed to exercise, almost like the Navy SEALs or Army Rangers who live in their houses with their families—as long as the country is peaceful. When danger presents itself, these highly trained military personnel are "called up" to carry out missions that will ultimately strengthen our country. The heat shock proteins react similarly, carrying out the mission of strengthening our bodies following exercise, then returning to their dormant state. These proteins are made of specific building blocks called amino acids.[17]

An illustrative example is seen in figure 18, the actual amino acid sequence of heat shock protein 90. Notice in the second part of the figure that the great majority of these proteins are comprised of the amino acids lysine and glutamic acid (their single-letter symbols in biochemistry-speak are K and E, respectively). In order to support this system of recovery, it will again be important to add these sources as supplements to our diet. Lysine-rich foods include roasted turkey, legumes (beans) like kidney beans and lentils, and—guess what catching point partici-

17 All proteins are made of specific building blocks called amino acids. That is, each protein in our body has a very specific job and is therefore structured specifically for that job based on its sequence of amino acids.

pants—soy beans! How's that for two birds with one stone. Foods rich in glutamic acid are grilled chicken, eggs, and—shut the front door—soy! Boy, we are really establishing a theme here now. Please read on.

Amino Acid Sequence HSP90

MPEETQTQDQPMEEEEVETFAFQAEIAQIMSLINTFYSNKEIFLRELISNSSDAIDKIRYESLTDP
DKLDSGKELHINLIPNKQDRTLTIVDTGIGMTKADLINNLGTIAKSGTKAFMEALQAGADISMI
GQFGVGFYSAYLVAEKVTVITKHNKKEQYAWESSAGGSFTVRTDTGEPMGRGTKVILHLKED
QTEYLEERRIKEIVKKHSQFIGYPITLFVEKERDKEVSDDEAEEKEDKEEEKEKEEKESEDKPEIED
VGSDEEEEKKDGOKKKKKKIKEKYIDQEELNKTKPIWTRNPDDITNEEYGEFYKSLTNDWEDH
LAVKHFSVEGQLEFRALLFVPRRAPFDLFENRKKKNNIKLYNEEYGEFYKSLTNDWEDHLAVK
HFSVEGQLEFRALLFVPRRAPFDLFENRKKKNNIKLYVRRVFIMDNCEELIPEYLNFIRGVVDSE
DLPLNISREMLQQSKILKVIRKNLVKKCLELFTELAEDKENYKKFYEQFSKNIKLGIHEDSQNRKK
LSELLRYYTSASGDEMVSLKDYCTRMKENQKHIYYITGETKDQVANSAFVERLRKHGLEVIYMI
EPIDEYCVQQLKEFEGKTLVSVTKEGLELPEDEEEKKQEEKKTKFENLCKMKDILEKKVEKVVVS
NRLVTSPCCIVTSTYGWTANMERIMKAQALRDNSTMGMAAKKHLEINPDHSIIETLRQKAEA
DKNDKSVKDLVILLYETALLSSGFSLEDPQTHANRIYRMIKLGLGIDEDDPTADDTSAAVTEEM
PPLEGDDDTSRMEEVD

Amino Acid Sequence HSP90

MPEETQTQDQPMEEEEVETFAFQAEIAQIMSLINTFYSNKEIFLRELISNSSDAIDKIRYESLTDP
DKLDSGKELHINLIPNKQDRTLTIVDTGIGMTKADLINNLGTIAKSGTKAFMEALQAGADISMI
GQFGVGFYSAYLVAEKVTVITKHNKKEQYAWESSAGGSFTVRTDTGEPMGRGTKVILHLKED
QTEYLEERRIKEIVKKHSQFIGYPITLFVEKERDKEVSDDEAEEKEDKEEEKEKEEKESEDKPEIED
VGSDEEEEKKDGOKKKKKKIKEKYIDQEELNKTKPIWTRNPDDITNEEYGEFYKSLTNDWEDH
LAVKHFSVEGQLEFRALLFVPRRAPFDLFENRKKKNNIKLYNEEYGEFYKSLTNDWEDHLAVK
HFSVEGQLEFRALLFVPRRAPFDLFENRKKKNNIKLYVRRVFIMDNCEELIPEYLNFIRGVVDSE
DLPLNISREMLQQSKILKVIRKNLVKKCLELFTELAEDKENYKKFYEQFSKNIKLGIHEDSQNRKK
LSELLRYYTSASGDEMVSLKDYCTRMKENQKHIYYITGETKDQVANSAFVERLRKHGLEVIYMI
EPIDEYCVQQLKEFEGKTLVSVTKEGLELPEDEEEKKQEEKKTKFENLCKMKDILEKKVEKVVVS
NRLVTSPCCIVTSTYGWTANMERIMKAQALRDNSTMGMAAKKHLEINPDHSIIETLRQKAEA
DKNDKSVKDLVILLYETALLSSGFSLEDPQTHANRIYRMIKLGLGIDEDDPTADDTSAAVTEEM
PPLEGDDDTSRMEEVD

Figure 18. Actual amino acid sequence of human heat shock protein 90. The preponderance of lysine and glutamic acid warrant nutritional support during exercise program participation.

Selenium and Molybdenum

These are minerals that act against the reactive oxygen species generated during exercise. They are so effective in doing so that they are considered to have anticancer properties. In lay terms, these minerals are so effective against the little bouncing sour balls that damage our cells that they may be able to prevent cancer and are being incorporated as anticancer dietary supplements and even as part of new drugs aimed at controlling the development and growth of cancer. You need them to clear out the collateral damage caused by your exercise and to perform instrumental metabolic functions. Specifically, selenium and molybdenum function to adjust your metabolic rate in response to/as part of underlying restructuring in response to exercise. They are found in organ meats (liver, and so on), chicken, dark-green leafy vegetables, onions, garlic, and mushrooms.[145–147]

Chinese Walnuts

Any walnuts, really.[18] Walnuts contain a unique mixture of polyunsaturated fats and proteins. As a result, they do several things critical to your recovery. They burn slowly, which allows you to have a longer-lasting energy source. They contain plant proteins, which supply amino acids necessary for your transformation. And they have been shown to decrease the levels of circulating lipids (fats), lower risk for cardiovascular disease, and increase metabolism. Ultimately they tip you toward that selective digestion and storage pattern that will optimize your muscle/fat ratio. Moreover, they are rich in antioxidants, which may also prevent cancer and certainly aid in exercise recovery. Finally, for even the most pragmatic among us, they have been shown to make you feel less hungry, eat less, lose weight, *and literally live longer.*[148–150] Add them in.

Fish

Fish is a superfood.[147, 151–153] Fish contains omega-3 fatty acids, protein, vitamins, and minerals. It is a veritable gold mine of materials for transformation, restructuring, anti-inflammation effects, and recovery. It can also help your memory, make you feel better, and protect your

---

18 Do not eat walnuts if you are allergic to them or any potential nut ingredient or any possible component of any dish that may contain nuts or walnuts.

heart. Cold-water, wild, and fresh fish are best. Remember, though—we are adding these in at this point, not replacing other foods in your diet with them.[19]

Garlic

You may have heard this one before in the setting of heart disease. The same mechanism responsible for that effect, "scavenging reactive oxygen species," is beautifully suited for our purposes—and again, as an added bonus, prevents cancer. And diabetes. And arthritis. Garlic works after it's crushed by creating an enzyme (a protein) that absorbs (technically called "reducing") these damaging species. The same little buggers that bounce around and damage your DNA (leading to cancer) also damage your muscles, heart, and recovery scaffold. Sending crushed garlic through the digestive tract is like rolling a sticky ball of tape through lint. The garlic will reduce the reactive oxygen species on the way through, rendering them harmless and clearing the way for internal restructuring.[154, 155]

Protein Simple Carb Mix

This is an age-old known recovery element. It has stood the test of time, there are physiological explanations for its utility, and it is simple to add in. Within 45 minutes of any exercise session, the body is crazily gathering wood.[156–158] Remember, the body is looking to survive and adapt (it really doesn't care if you look good, except in that looking good might help you get sex, which will lead to species survival drive—but that's another topic), so it immediately begins the adaptation survival sequence when it determines the exercise assault has safely passed.

Consider the tanning response. The brain doesn't want you to get cancer from ultraviolet radiation, so when you go on vacation and lie out in the sun, it responds. As per our established theme, the brain says, "Well, if we are going to have to do this task, now we've got to adapt." So the brain sends signals to cells in the skin to dump a molecule called melanin, which will protect you from this exposure. There are many examples of brain-driven, molecule-mediated stimulus/adaptation phenomena like this, but I think you get the point.

---

19 Do not eat fish if you are allergic to it or any potential fish ingredient or any possible component of any dish that may contain fish or aquatic animal parts, or if you are pregnant or nursing a small child.

To capitalize on the initial wood-gathering phase of the adaptation response, you must load up and provide the body with exactly what it is looking for. It is looking for simple carbohydrates to store as glycogen for energy in order to survive the next assault, and protein to build muscle for the tasks.[20] The simplest way to accomplish this is to pour 20 grams of protein powder into a bottle of Gatorade (whey protein is fine, though there are specific recovery mixes too). Shake it up and drink it within the 45-minute window. The ideal thing would be to consume a relatively large fish and potato meal within that 45 minutes, or even steak and rice, cavatelli and meatballs, barbeque chicken and a baked potato, or a peanut butter sandwich with banana. The key is, eat protein and carbohydrates within 45 minutes. If your options are limited because of work, family, time constraints, etc., drink the Gatorade-protein mix. If you live on a private island with cooks and servants, eat salmon and pesto or filet mignon and twice-baked potatoes. Just eat and get full within that 45 minutes.[21]

For the data hounds and perfectionists, there is the notion of a leucine trigger to make this better.[37, 159] Exercise, particularly resistance exercise, opens a particular gate in the muscle right after the workout that streams in substances for new synthesis. That is, for a brief time following an exercise session, the muscle is open for new ideas—for restructuring.[160] It has been shown that the most welcome of the amino acids through this gate is leucine, and moreover, that leucine sets off, or "triggers," the construction of a new framework. Essentially a door is open and—if present—a whole bunch of leucine will be collected as bricks and wood for transformation. The end product will burn more calories for you, make you stronger and healthier, and increase your ability to exercise. It has also been shown that replenishment of fluids positively influences this sequence further, so if you're so inclined to improve this approach, a leucine supplement and the larger-size Gatorade for your whey mix would be ideal here.[161]

On several occasions I have had patients ask me, "Why don't I eat nothing after my workout and thereby have a negative calorie balance? Aren't I just putting right back the 400 calories I just burned?" Legitimate question, if we are still thinking old school: that we are going to

20 In the long run, this is super-duper important because muscles are great metabolizers.

21 An important point here is that if you go the Gatorade-protein powder route, eat a solid meal as soon as possible afterward. You want tons of wood to be available in these few hours post-exercise.

be able to burn more calories than we take in to lose weight. In the new school, though, you are exercising to change your inner structure in order to ultimately burn more calories at rest and improve your existing exercise capacity (which is really worthless at this point; sorry—tough love) to a point that will allow you to burn real amounts of calories and follow demanding exercise programs. During these 45 minutes, your body is trying to do exactly that by sweeping up nutrients to be stored as glycogen and to serve as building blocks for muscle transformation. If you don't make available those nutrients, then yes, your body may turn and suck some fat cells out in order to try and get nutrients—which will result in a leptin surge (see chapter 3) that will cross your eyes with hunger pangs so that you will ultimately eat to replace your fat. So good question, but don't try it.

Raw Vegetables

Fifteen at a time. Before a meal. This is not a trick. The reason you need to eat these before your meal is not to trick you into eating less (though that is not a bad idea, down the road); at this point it is to prevent you from getting full on other foods and *not* eating them. We need vegetables for recovery for a variety of reasons, the two most important of which are natural vitamins and minerals and the digestive properties of fiber. Vitamins and minerals all have specific functions in the body, many of which were discovered when people lost access to them (the functions, I mean, not the vitamins). The scope of vitamin and mineral function is way beyond this book—but suffice it to say that they too are molecules and function as workers to build the scaffold. For example, potassium functions in muscle contraction, nerve impulse transduction, and cell membrane integrity. Iron functions in oxygen transport, and so on. Through complex interactions, we need vitamins and minerals to recover, and we need fiber to digest them. They are the workers that construct the scaffold and arrange the molecules to our advantage.[22]

Even better, grow vegetables yourself. The pesticides and chemicals applied to store-bought vegetables are potentially carcinogenic (i.e., they may be linked to cancer). In fact, any mass-produced food for public consumption is likely to have undergone some "processing," which in

22 Synthetic vitamins in supplements probably don't function the same way. The reasons for this are likely related to their modification between when you ingest them and when they get to the site of action. There is much controversy around this topic, but no one argues the value of natural vitamins and minerals, so let's just stick with what we know for sure.

general is detrimental to your health. Of course, most of us don't live on farms and must function within our limits, but if you have the time, room, or interest, I recommend growing as many fresh vegetables in your yard as possible (figure 19).

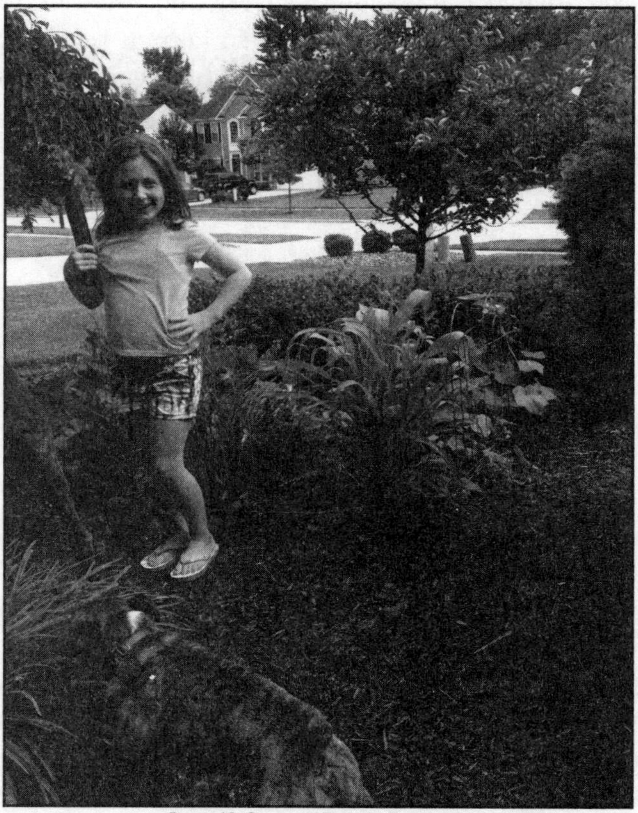

Figure 19. Grace and Tank the Pug showcase a suburban garden.

WATER

Osmoregulation. Yup, osmoregulation. The idea that the body regulates its water composition. You've heard many times that so much of the human body is water, which is true—but the real issue is balance. Balance of the body's water stores occurs across cell membranes as determined by a gradient, conveniently called the osmotic gradient. The kidneys are the main regulators of this balance, and they do so by (oversimplification alert) measuring the concentration of ions in the blood. That is, if things are too concentrated, the kidneys send messages to drink, or pull water from the cells. In ideal conditions, which is what we want, and why water is included here, the cells are surrounded by a dilute system. You create a dilute system by drinking lots of water. You want a dilute system because the body will balance this out by creating more urine and detoxifying the system along the way. Lactic acid and other metabolites created by exercise may hinder your recovery, and you want your kidneys to clean them out. Moreover, the cells then keep as much water as they want for their own scaffold building instead of having it sucked out into the bloodstream because your system is too concentrated. One gallon in a day, ideally spring water.[23, 24]

Vinegar

Cell uptake regulation. Insulin is a hormone in the body whose job it is (in part) to get things into cells, particularly glucose. This is important because anything that you put in to your body is only useful if it ultimately gets inside the relevant cells, be it muscle cells, heart cells, brain cells, or other. Its mechanisms of action and interplay with other functions of the body are exceedingly complex. For us, we would like to affect that interplay in a way that ultimately leads to *efficient* utilization of nutrients. That is to say that we are interested at this point in the building-block properties of the food we eat, in targeted protein synthesis. Several studies have shown that vinegar intake may positively affect glycemic index, satiety, overall glucose levels in the blood, and cholesterol levels. Add two tablespoons of vinegar to two cups of water and drink before the last meal of the day in order to target the body's plan for the nutrients contained in the food you eat before bed.[162–165]

Chromium

Obesity physicians prescribe chromium to curb sugar cravings. This is something you can supplement to in part block the brain from sending out "eat some sugar" messages.[166–168] It does this by combining with proteins in the body to form a complex called chromodulin. Without getting too far into the biochemistry, chromodulin binds to places where glucose (sugar) binds. This tells the body that you have enough circulating sugar, and the brain then backs off its survival search for sugar. Broccoli, grape juice, black pepper, and thyme are the best sources.

23 The one caveat to this is don't drink so much that you can't sleep because you are urinating. Choose sleep over water if it comes to that.

24 Not *every* day. *Per* day. This will be one of the program options for a given day.

Active Recovery

The term "active recovery" is meant to differentiate this change accelerant with the changes that occur during sleep (passive recovery). These are things that you can do with your body to encourage and nurture change and recovery.

For much of this book, we have discussed the real physical connections and molecular messengers that travel between the brain and body—and have stressed how important this network will be to recovery. First, it is imperative that you recognize these signals from the brain to the body and react accordingly. Second, *you can induce the mind to accelerate recovery and protect you on your journey.*

The classic example of this is visualization, a technique employed for years to perfect physical performances—which can now be defined as specific reorganization of the brain molecules through imagery. The great news is, this process is enhanced by exercise.[45, 169–171] To be clear, the quiet reflection on one's physical goals actually changes the composition of the brain matter, which results in positive feedback in an antegrade direction (from the brain, out) to the body, which has been shown to positively affect physical performance, anxiety, insomnia, pain, circulation, inflammation, and—you guessed it—obesity. Professor Ann Taylor and her coauthors state clearly that "it has become increasingly clear that bidirectional ('top-down and bottom up') interactions between the brain and peripheral tissues, including the cardiovascular and immune systems, contribute to both mental and physical health."[172] So how can we take advantage of this network during recovery? As follows.

Yoga, Meditation, and Focused Imagery

To be consistent, we are looking for actual, identifiable, physical changes that follow these activities, not the prophecy of your Aunt Helen who's enamored with her Pilates instructor or your friend Sally who goes to hot yoga. For this we return to the reactive oxygen species (the bouncing sour balls). It is commonly known that exercise creates these damaging little guys, and that they cause us problems with recovery and make us feel crappy.[92, 173] All three of these interventions (yoga, meditation, and imagery) have been shown to reduce the levels of reactive oxygen species and the damage that goes with them, thereby improving physical recovery and protecting humans from disease.[174–177] Moreover, these practices positively affect the nervous system tone such that quality of life is improved, heart rate and blood pressure are decreased, glucose tolerance is controlled, and disease relapse rates in stem-cell recipients are lowered.[178]

There are many types of yoga and many types of meditation, and focused imagery is a made-up term meant to encompass progressive muscle relaxation through object and/or breathing focus to traditional visualization of you shooting foul shots (or hitting tennis balls, or swinging kettlebells, or whatever). The benefit of each is the exploitation of the mind-body nexus to induce those molecules that will result in organ transformation. Taking part in these activities in between workouts will be the difference between this program and others you have failed. It will direct the body toward recovery from stress deregulation.[179, 180]

The central theme of yoga is to join the mind and body. It is a discipline that focuses on physical postures and meditative techniques in order to improve flexibility, strength, balance, awareness, and peace. The simplest of yoga techniques can be distilled to a lying posture, with a blanket and pillow positioned underneath your back and you faceup. This exercise takes place somewhere quiet: in a private room, in the park under a tree, etc. For 20 or so minutes, you will observe your breath. Track it as you inhale, feel it as your rib cage and belly expand, listen as it makes its way out when you exhale. Imagine that the pure oxygen you bring in flows through your body, between the muscle fibers, to your toes, and through each chamber of your heart as it brings purity to your body. Know that each breath brings with it snow-white clarity and change. Each inflow makes its way through every area of your body, bringing with it the breeze of change, and each outflow means the exit of everything that has been holding you back. You've got the secret to transformation now. You've set it in motion with your physical exercise, and now you are directing your body to change, to adjust, to rid itself of toxins and sludge with each exhalation—to make you strong.

What I've described above can itself increase your exercise capacity, rid you of poisons, make you healthier, and even change your gene expression.[177, 181–183] It also points to a larger concept that is relevant for catching point participants called mindfulness. Certainly we are all drawn to the future by the hope of better things. Bright prospects for our children, promotions for us, vacations, new houses, better bodies, and so on. Like most things, though, this draw can be all-consuming and can potentially debunk our efforts to get there. More specifically, a section of our nervous system—called sympathetic tone—can be increased by a low-level anxiety because we don't have this better body (or promotion, or acceptance for our child to a college) just yet. Although that anxiety can drive you in a positive direction, it can also cross a line and become counterproductive. That increased tone can block the reparative changes we are after.

> We are all drawn to the future by the hope of better things. Bright prospects for our children, promotions for us, vacations, new houses, better bodies, and so on.

Mindfulness seeks to find happiness and peace *in the process*, not in the end product. For most of this program you will not look like your desired end product, so if you use that as your measure of happiness each day, you will be repeatedly disappointed for some time. Use the presence or absence *of progress* as your measure. Know that you are making changes and are on your way. Be mindful of that instead of the distance you have to go. As originally written by Thich Nhat Hanh and reproduced by yoga instructor Christine Felstead:

> If while washing dishes, we think only of the cup of tea that awaits us, thus hurrying to get the dishes out of the way as if they were a nuisance...we are not alive during the time we are washing the dishes. If we can't wash the dishes, the chances are we won't be able to drink our tea either...we will only be thinking of other things...thus we are sucked away into the future, and we are incapable of actually living one minute of life.[184,185]

Mindfulness seeks a higher level of peace, well-being, and contentment with a process that is pleasant, but for the purposes of this book it should be sought in order to allow body transformation to occur. Plainly said, do your best to throw out any anxious feelings or discontent you have because of your current physical state. Find peace in your pursuit.

You are doing the right thing, you are on the right track, and you should be glad at the end of each of these days. That gladness will grease the wheels of your transformation.

A much better alternative for that anxiety is the meditation strategy of visualization. Using the same sequence as described for yogic breathing above, find a peaceful, quiet place and initiate the breathing focus as above. However, after five minutes switch your focus from the breathing to your ideal body. Imagine your hips, belly, and thighs (or your abs, arms, and quads) in perfect form. Construct the ideal you in your mind down to every last detail. Focus on your slender moves, your curves or cuts, and your skin tone. Spend 15 minutes working out in your mind with this ideal person. Allow yourself to *know* that this is where you are headed now, and that you have time to get there. Define your goal with a picture in your mind and allow yourself to believe it is a reality. Feel happy because you've found the way there. Imagine it with the same confidence you would dream about a beach vacation you've planned next year, or the way you counted down to Christmas as a kid. You know it's coming, you can't make it get here any faster, but you anticipate that it will happen—and that it will be awesome.

Visualization can segue and overlap with guided imagery and progressive muscle relaxation. For example, during these visualizations, flex the muscles involved with your picture. Tighten your abs, for example, as you examine each detail of the pose in your mind. Hold the flex pose for several seconds, then release and relax.[25] Next, do the same with your quadriceps, hamstrings, and so on. This sequence is called progressive muscle relaxation, and it has been shown time and time again to prevent injury, hasten recovery, and improve overall health.[186–188] With or without linking your visualization images, tense your muscles for several seconds one at a time, beginning with your neck and ending with your toes, resting in between to complete the sequence. Finally, guided imagery then takes your ideal self from your visualization exercise and walks him or her through the peaceful, happy, fun existence that you seek. See yourself relaxing on a hammock or going to the gym or shopping for produce, as beautiful and fit as you can dream it. Feel your muscle movements during the imagery, flex, and relax—thereby linking mind and body and moving toward your goal.

25 Don't forget, all of this is happening in the privacy of your own mind, in a quiet room or under a tree where you are alone. So if any of it sounds silly or embarrassing, please get over that. This is what you have been missing, and these techniques result in real changes that are observable and measurable in the long run.

There are other types of yoga and other types of meditation. For example, creating a music playlist for your workouts or for your quiet times is a form of focus therapy. Pursue them all; learn about them. Part of the action options/workout options for the program will suggest reaching out to participate or learn about these techniques formally when you are ready. The direction itself is kinetic in that once that first step is taken and you declare yourself present, there are a multitude of other benefits that may follow—including a social pull toward those groups of happy healthy livers we've watched from afar for so long. Consider it as an option for contributing to your well of positivity (see chapter 11).

Another option (favored by the author of this book and program) along the spectrum of meditative techniques are daily reflections. This can be done in one of several ways, all of which are valuable. For Christians, the book *Jesus Calling* contains reflections for every day of the year—drawing, of course, from the role of God in our daily lives. These reflections accomplish a multitude of things, from defining a few moments of peace and silence while you read them to grounding your perspective in daily life. Keeping your mind tethered (like a hot air balloon anchored to the ground) is important during this process, for it will aid in maintaining a pace you can stay with for 84 days. Remember, we are stressing and adapting—do everything you can to keep your mind sane during the adaptation phases. Resist the temptation of your mind to stray from the program. These focus points will help do that. There are websites with daily reflections and inspirations, apps that will send you quotes each day, and so on.

Alternatively, write down in a log your thoughts from the day. Reflect on where you are in your journey and what external factors may be influencing or distracting you. Consider this your logbook during a treacherous journey from which you cannot escape. An 84-day tour of duty that requires you to be alert for survival. Write down how your homesickness and your fear threaten to distract you but that you can't give in—because you've got only X number of days to go, and you want to hug your loved ones and put this behind you when it's over. Recognize and put in print any potential derailing forces in your life. It will be like shining a spotlight on someone sneaking up to rob you, and it will tighten the knot on your tether.

The Relaxation Sequence

This sequence is designed to be performed on the second day following a workout. That is, if you work out on Monday, this is for Wednesday. Twenty-four hours after a workout your body has gathered wood, synthesized protein, and initiated changes in response to your exercise. It's the body reacting to what it interprets as a new thing it may be called on to do. The brain and body are efficient, though, and unfortunately for us will do the bare minimum to repair organs and prepare for a potential additional strike in the form of exercise. I mean, let's face it, up until now the odds have been long that your body would undergo *another* round of exercise, and even longer that the next round would be something for which the body should prepare! So the body builds the minimum scaffold it thinks necessary, figuring not to expend too much energy on this issue that is most likely temporary.

Catching point participants, though, need to send the message to continue and increase the amount of changes because you need to be prepared for additional and progressive rounds of exercise down the road. For this reason, at 24 to 48 hours we engage in the relaxation sequence, which is static stretching, followed by hot tub time, then cold-water swimming.[26] Specifically, the static stretch time should include 15- to 20-second stretches of the calves, hamstrings, quadriceps and hip flexors, groin musculature, shoulders, and neck, followed by 8 to 10 minutes of direct hot tub massage (sit in front of one of the bubblers or under the falls), then two laps of cold-water slow-extension swimming, then repeat. The logic behind this sequence is that static stretching resets the length of muscle fibers. What this means is that you are forcing your body to reset its molecular structure to adapt to increasing levels of exercise.

To illustrate, imagine that your brain has decided to build a canvas to catch people who are jumping from a burning building. The brain is not entirely sure if you are really ever going to use this thing, so it gathers some spring metal and rubber and assembles one that is 2 feet by 2 feet. During the relaxation sequence, you stretch the canvas to 10 feet by 10 feet, forcing the brain to resize the metal portion to fit and accommodate more jumpers. You increase the capacity of the canvas. Likewise, you are

---

26 The actual sequence is sauna or steam room time (including static stretching in the heat), hot tub time, cold-water swimming, and back to the heat, the hot tub, the pool, and done. Unfortunately, I cannot advise anyone to partake in this because of the potential adverse health effects of the heat. Consult with your doctor before partaking in any of this, but particularly before you get in a sauna or steam room.

increasing the capacity of your body to handle exercise through the relaxation sequence. As an added bonus, I am also willing to bet that you will sleep better that night.

Massage, Active Release, and/or Self-Myofascial Release

This is the relaxation sequence on steroids. I include these tools because they are supremely effective but realize also that they are time consuming. Time-consuming activities can speed your progress toward the cliff (from chapter 5), so you have to be careful. *If* your schedule allows for these activities during the 48 hours following your workout, then I recommend you try them. All three require either the assistance of an expert or self-education, but they have great returns. Massage requires no explanation and often can be combined with mental and/or spiritual recovery as well. Active release is a massage technique that requires training on the part of the therapist and involves stabilizing one insertion point of your muscle while dragging the hand down the muscle in order to free the fascia. Self-myofascial release is the use of foam rollers to accomplish the same goal.

The logic behind these techniques is to combat the overkill of recovery, a situation comparable to allergies. People with allergies have an immune response to something (pollen, peanut butter, bee stings) that is way out of proportion to normal. The immune system normally recognizes a foreign substance, like bacteria, and launches an attack. In the setting of allergies, this attack is either so intense that it damages the body, is launched against something harmless, or both. Either way, the response has to be tempered to protect the body and brain. Similarly, the recovery response to exercise can go too far and be damaging, especially to untrained folks. The assault on the body that induces the signals for recovery that this entire book is centered around can also elicit some unwanted inflammation—much like allergies. In this setting, that response will result in muscle "tightening," which we combat primarily with the relaxation sequence. It can also result in a phenomenon called fascial tightening. Fascia is like clear plastic wrap around and between your muscles. If it gets inflamed, it can get sticky and limit your movement. These techniques bust up that stickiness and release the "glued" fascia from your muscles so that you can continue to expand the canvas.

The support of the logic is found in the scientific literature, the most important of which (in my opinion) was done at Emory University.[189] Massage was shown to decrease cortisol (the stress hormone) as well as decrease inflammatory mediators—attenuating the collateral damage that goes along with those markers. These effects are likely to be more pronounced post-exercise. Beyond this study, massage has been shown to benefit symptoms related to back pain, anxiety, depression, asthma, cancer, and substance abuse.[189–191]

Compression Devices

These devices support recovery through improved circulation.[192, 193] They may also provide anti-inflammatory effects and mechanical support. The options for use of compression devices are empiric (meaning wearing compression stockings to increase blood flow in the absence of any injury or soreness) or directed (meaning that you wear a Copper Fit or some such device for your sore elbow or knee). Most studies have demonstrated improved recovery, better ability to exercise and perform tasks, and potential mechanical support for injuries with these devices.

Cold Immersion

Therapeutic cold immersion originated from attempts to slow or halt the inflammatory process following injury. It has since been extrapolated to a condition called delayed onset muscle soreness (DOMS). The basic idea is similar to the above description of fascial thickening—that microtrauma to the muscles results in changes in surrounding electrolytes and mediators of inflammation and creates by-products of energy "burning," one of which is called lactic acid. Now, the presence of soreness following a workout (thanks to the lactic acid) is an indicator that there was trauma to the system. This is what we want, though, right? This is a delicate dance, but to be succinct: soreness is fine. Cold immersion pools or cold-water swimming affect soreness incidentally. We are interested in the increased blood flow, decreased carbon dioxide, and accelerated recovery associated with these techniques.[194–196]

The Soul

Books have been written on how the soul and/or mind relate to the body through healing, health, and wellness. Even more has been written on the subject in isolation. This book even describes the mind-body connection and how it can be exploited to accomplish your goals. In the setting of reorganizing your body using exercise as the stimulus, nurturing and attention to the soul are powerful tools.

Now, before you skip this part because it sounds too touchy-feely, let me assure you that the mind-body connection has resulted in documented, objective events. Emotional distress has been shown to weaken the immune system, disrupt the gastrointestinal system, interrupt sleep, cause high blood pressure, worsen pain, and much more. The flip side of this coin is that emotional nurturing has been shown to decrease cortisol levels (a nasty survival-based hormone that breaks down muscle, stores fat, and many other bad things), enhance sleep, decrease hospital stays, relieve pain, and change people's overall perception of well-being.

There are several schools of thought regarding the mechanism by which the mind-body connection results in molecular reorganization, but few disagree that it happens. In fact, businesses spend millions of dollars each year to improve the performance of executives through integration of hope, mindfulness, and renewal. In that arena they are less concerned with the specific molecules that change, but they measure outcome variables such as productivity and perception of well-being. They are exploiting the mind-body connection in reverse—realizing that the connection is there, they are stressing relaxation, renewal, and so on in an attempt to affect the neural signals back to the brain for intellectual results. Likewise, music therapists are now employed by hospitals, as are art therapists, guided imagery experts, tai chi instructors, and religious liaisons. Medical experts know there is value to nurturing the mind-body connection, and businesses see the return on their investment in this arena. In this setting we aren't recovering from illness or seeking renewal after 100-hour workweeks; we are accelerating the process of molecular reorganization and physical change after carefully timed and designed rounds of exercise, with the intent of increasing our capacity to enjoy diet and exercise and ultimately meet our fitness goals.

The theory in this section translates in the overall program as progressive muscle relaxation, mind relaxation, guided imagery, relaxation breathing, and prayer. Alternatives include other types of meditation, tai chi, nature walks, positive reflection, and group reinforcement.

Here are two additional real-life options: think about it during drive time, and pay attention to your reserve. To begin with, whenever you are driving by yourself, focus on your body. Think about the changes that are happening inside you as a result of your last workout, your rest, and your positive progress. Focus on any muscle soreness or sign that your body is changing. Link that feeling to peace. Know that you've planted a seed and it is growing now—and take pride in that. Focus on your breathing. Take a few deep breaths and know that your lungs are cleaner and healthier because of the program you've joined. Relax your feet. Only you know what is happening inside your body. It's like a secret you have from the world. Your progress is ongoing. You're switching castes. Be happy about that.

Second, always be attentive to your reserve. Imagine if something unexpected were to happen in your life tomorrow, like a relative came to live with you or your car broke down. Would that tip you over the edge? If the answer is yes, then your reserve is poor. You should always have some gas in the tank; otherwise you can't recover. Imagine that you never run your life at greater than 90 percent capacity. You always have 10 percent of your energy stored away. This will keep you from running in overdrive, which prevents recovery, accelerates disease, makes you age faster, keeps you fat, and so on. So two or three times a day, take two or three quiet minutes and assess your reserve. If you feel like you're running close to empty, take a nap. Have lunch in the park. Go for a walk. Say some prayers. Go to church. Read this book. Re-center yourself. In fact, the essence of this book is to shift your focus from the workouts and the diet to the changes that occur during peaceful states. This should be your first priority during these 84 days. This program absolutely, categorically depends on your rest and tranquility.

The Recoveries

The recoveries are listed below, one per box. Choose from these as you progress toward the program (explained in Chapter 11).

The Recipes

These will also count as your recovery options. These are 15 select recipes that we intend to serve up as the first food-related amalgamation.[27] Remember, these contain the nutrients you want to have during recovery to fire up your metabolism. Add these meals in on days you can.

27 To "amalgamate" is to combine or unite into one form. It is the perfect way to put this. We want to smoothly combine these habits, these foods, these recoveries into your life. Amalgamation.

MEDITERRANEAN QUINOA SALAD

Ingredients

- 2 cups chicken broth
- 1 clove garlic, chopped
- 1 cup quinoa
- 2 large chicken breasts, cooked and cut into bite-sized pieces
- ½ red onion, chopped
- 1 green pepper, chopped
- ½ cup kalamata olives, pitted
- ½ cup crumbled feta
- ¼ cup chopped parsley
- ¼ cup chopped chives

Dressing

- ⅔ cup lemon juice
- 1 tablespoon balsamic vinegar
- ¼ cup olive oil

In a medium-size pan, bring to boil the chicken broth, garlic, and quinoa. Cover and simmer about 20 minutes, until the water is absorbed. In a large bowl, combine the chicken, onion, pepper, olives, feta, parsley, and chives. Mix in cooked quinoa. Combine dressing ingredients and mix into chicken mixture. Serve hot or cold.

CHILI

Ingredients

- 1–1½ lbs. lean ground beef
- 2 15-ounce cans black beans, rinsed
- 1 large onion, chopped
- 2 tablespoons chili powder
- 1 large green pepper, chopped
- 1 teaspoon garlic, minced
- 1 15-ounce can petite diced tomatoes
- 1 teaspoon cumin
- 1 teaspoon salt and pepper
- ½ cup barbeque sauce

Brown the beef in a large skillet, adding some of the spices to flavor the meat while its cooking. Drain excess grease. Combine all ingredients in a large pot, bring to boil, then cover and simmer. Stir every 15 minutes for approximately 1 hour, adjusting spices to taste.

LETTUCE WRAPS

Ingredients

- Romaine lettuce leaves
- 1 lb. lean ground beef or shredded chicken
- 1 package taco seasoning
- ½ onion, chopped
- ½ cup black olives, sliced
- Shredded cheddar to taste
- Cilantro and crushed corn chips

Cook the beef or chicken, add taco seasoning to taste. Place small amount of meat onto romaine lettuce and add other ingredients to taste. Top with your favorite salsa or Avocado Ranch Dressing.

AVOCADO RANCH DRESSING

Ingredients

- 1 avocado, pitted
- ½ cup sour cream or plain Greek yogurt
- ¼ cup milk
- 1 tablespoon lemon juice
- 1½ teaspoon rice vinegar
- 3 cloves garlic, minced
- 2 tablespoons parsley, chopped
- ¼ teaspoon salt

Mash avocado, then mix in sour cream/yogurt. Mix in milk, then add other ingredients one at a time. Chill for 30 minutes.

ASIAGO CHICKEN SAUSAGE

Ingredients

- 4 links Asiago chicken sausage
- ½ green and red pepper, cut into bite-size pieces
- ½ red onion, cut into wedges
- 1 tablespoon olive oil
- 1 box rice, brown or white

In a large skillet, add oil and cook peppers and onions until crisp, about 3 minutes. Broil sausage on high for approximately 4 minutes, then turn and broil another 4 minutes until browned. Cut sausages into bite-size slices and stir into pepper/onion. Serve over rice.

CRISPY BRAZIL NUT BARS

Ingredients

- 1 cup cashew butter
- 1 cup Brazil nuts
- 1 cup honey
- 1 cup sliced almonds
- 1 cup flaxseed
- ½ cup dried cranberries
- 1 teaspoon ground cinnamon
- 2 cups Rice Krispies

Lightly coat a 9" x 13" baking dish with nonstick cooking spray. In a food processor, grind Brazil nuts until fine and place in a large mixing bowl. Add the almonds, flaxseeds, cranberries, cinnamon, and cereal to the bowl. In a large saucepan on the stove, combine the cashew butter and honey and heat until hot and bubbling. Transfer this mixture to the mixing bowl and mix together using a wooden spoon. Press mixture firmly into the baking dish. 5 minutes of cooling, cut into desired shapes.

EGG MUFFINS

Ingredients

- Chopped vegetables: broccoli, peppers, onions, carrots, etc. +/– cut sausage, ham, or crumbled bacon
- Eggs
- Shredded mozzarella or cheddar cheese
- 1% or skim milk

Grease a large cupcake pan and add your favorite chopped veggies or cut sausage, ham cubes, or cooked crumbled bacon until each cup is ▯ full. Mix 1 egg with a splash of milk and pour on top of filling. Bake at 425°F for approximately 15 to 20 minutes. Top with cheese.

THE MEGA SALAD

Ingredients

- Chopped romaine and baby spinach
- ½ cup chicken, chopped or shredded
- 1 hard-boiled egg
- ¼ cup broccoli, chopped
- ½ small avocado, pitted and chopped
- 1 green onion, chopped
- Green/red pepper, chopped
- 12 tablespoons sliced almonds
- 1–2 tablespoons dried cranberries or sliced grapes
- 5 cherry tomatoes
- Cucumber, chopped
- 3 tablespoons favorite dressing

Combine all ingredients, including dressing, in plastic bowl. Secure lid and shake well.

LEMON PEPPER GREEN BEANS AND ALMONDS

Ingredients

- 1 package frozen cut green beans
- ¼ cup sliced almonds
- 1 tablespoon butter
- 2 tablespoons lemon pepper

Cook beans per package directions. In a large skillet, melt butter and sauté almonds until browned, then add the lemon pepper and mix well. Stir in the beans to coat.

CHICKEN STIR-FRY

Ingredients

- 1 lb. cooked cubed chicken
- 1 green/red pepper, cut into bite-sized pieces
- 1 small red onion, cut into wedges
- 1 tablespoon olive oil
- ¼ cup fine chopped pineapple
- Soy sauce
- 1 box rice, brown or white

Heat oil and cook peppers and onions until crisp tender. Add pineapple and chicken and stir until heated. Drizzle with soy sauce or your favorite sauce. Serve over rice.

CHICKEN TORTILLA SOUP

Ingredients

- 1 lb. cooked shredded chicken
- 1 package taco seasoning
- 3 cups chicken broth
- 15-ounce petite diced tomatoes with chiles or jalapeños
- 1 small onion, chopped
- 8 ounces shredded Mexican-blend cheese
- ¼ cup cilantro or green onion, chopped

In a large pot, combine all ingredients except chicken and bring to a boil, then simmer for approximately 5 minutes. Add chicken and continue to simmer until heated. For thicker soup, combine ¼ cup cold water with 2 tablespoons cornstarch to make paste, add to soup, and bring to boil for 1 minute, stirring until thickened. Top the soup with cheese and cilantro or green onion.

BAKED GARLIC FRIES

Ingredients

- 2 russet potatoes, cut into wedges
- 1 tablespoon olive oil
- ¼ teaspoon salt and pepper
- ¼ teaspoon paprika
- 1 teaspoon garlic, powder or minced

Mix garlic and spices in oil, coat potatoes in mix, and place on foil-lined baking sheet. Bake at 400°F for 15 minutes. Turn potatoes and bake additional 15 minutes or until tender.

THE SLEEPER

Ingredients

- ½–1 lb. sliced roasted turkey
- ¼ cup cottage cheese
- 3 slices of white or whole-grain bread
- Tart cherry juice
- Paprika to taste

Toast bread, spread on cottage cheese, and sprinkle with paprika. Put the turkey next to the toasted bread on the plate for a real nice presentation. Couple this with cherry juice to drink. This meal is perfect for a late-night snack.

SOY STEW

Ingredients

- 2 tablespoons soybean oil
- 2 cups chopped onions
- 1 large green pepper, chopped
- 3 tablespoons soy flour
- 2 cans beef broth
- 1 fresh tomato, chopped
- 8 ounces frozen tofu, thawed
- 1 teaspoon ground cumin
- 1 teaspoon black pepper
- 1 pinch garlic powder
- 4 cups cooked rice or noodles

On medium-high heat, heat oil in large soup pot. Chop tofu. Add onions to pot and cook until slightly soft, about 2 to 3 minutes. Add soy flour and stir constantly as flour starts to brown, about 2 minutes. Add beef broth. Raise heat to high and stir to loosen any brown bits from flour. Add green pepper. Cover pot and bring to a boil, about 3 minutes. Add tomatoes and spices. Cover and boil until tender, about 3 to 4 minutes. Serve over rice or noodles.

CHRISTMAS EVE BACCALÀ

Ingredients

- ¼ cup extra-virgin olive oil
- 1 small onion
- ½ red pepper
- Crushed red hot pepper
- 2 cans crushed tomatoes
- 2 lbs. baccalà
- 1 pinch oregano
- 1 pinch parsley
- 1 pinch black pepper
- 1 pinch garlic powder
- Angel hair noodles

Soak baccalà in fresh water for 24 hours. In a medium saucepan, heat the olive oil over medium heat. Add onion and pepper and cook for 10 minutes. Add spices and tomatoes, then bring to a slow boil, stirring often. Add fish and simmer for 20 minutes. Serve over angel-hair pasta.

Recovery Interventions

Soy Shake and Nap
Have a soy protein shake today made with 1% or skim milk in the morning. Nap for 2 hours minimum. In a quiet room. In the afternoon. Recover. Relax. Rebuild.

Selenium and Molybdenum
Create a targeted antioxidant meal. It could include chicken, mushrooms, garlic, spinach. Provide your body that cleanup metabolism booster it craves in between workouts today. Eat this meal for dinner, then relax, sleep, recover.

Leucine Trigger and Hot Tub
Use this day to prepare for your next workout recovery trigger. Collect 2 Gatorades and whey and leucine supplements. Prepare them to be mixed and taken in immediately after your next workout. Spend 15 to 30 minutes in a hot tub or hot bath. Prepare. Recover. Plan. Relax.

Raw Vegetables +/– Fruit
Today consume a large bowl of raw vegetables with or without vinegar to taste before lunch and dinner: broccoli, cauliflower, carrots, cucumbers, celery, etc. Add some fruit to taste in between.

Water and Vinegar
Today take a shot (or a double shot) of white vinegar in the morning and before bed. Chase it with water. Consume 1 gallon of spring water throughout the day, preferably during the first two-thirds of the day.

Focused Imagery

Find 30 minutes today to engage in focused imagery. If you haven't read this section in chapter 9, use your 30 minutes to do that today. If you have, focus on your ideal self in a quiet environment down to the smallest detail while breathing deliberately and relaxing. CDs and downloads are available to help you with this as well. They can be used through headphones to guide you, but do not use your phone, as interruptions will diminish/ruin your experience here.

The Relaxation Sequence

If you haven't read this section in chapter 9, use 30 minutes to do that today. If you have, focus on conditioning your body to absorb more exercise and adapt. Stretch, relax, reset.

Massage, Active Release, or Self-Myofascial Release

Options for today: (1) get a traditional deep-muscle massage from a licensed sports therapy masseuse; (2) undergo active release therapy (ART) from a trained and certified practitioner; (3) use the foam roller for a self-myofascial release.

Lunasin and Soluble Fiber Cleanse

Today you are going to blunt your body's response to sugar and cleanse your digestive tract so you can adapt and be more efficient in your recoveries. During the day today, at any time consume **all** of the following separately (not at the same meal): two cups oatmeal made with 1% skim milk; two servings of either lima beans, kidney beans, or soy beans; and sweet potatoes.

The Snack Planner

Today, pack your snacks for the day in a sealable plastic container. Choose fruits, cereals, nut/pretzel mixes, vegetables, peanut butter, etc. Focus on what you eat as snacks, including the after-dinner snack. Plan. Learn. Evolve.

Recon

Today, explore outside options. Think about where you want to be at the end of this journey, and look for something you may imagine doing: spinning, yoga, CrossFit, running clubs, etc. Consider which day next week you can join a sample class. Look ahead to swapping one day out for a structured, outside-the-home class. Don't buy a membership—make a plan to try one class. Alternatively, find a hill or stadium stairs to do your next walk. Look for a bike trail or a biking team or rowing club. Something that gets you out and physically active. Build options for the future.

20 Minutes

Today, try the 20 minutes tool. No need to limit your food intake—you are harnessing fuel and satisfaction for your next workout. But for today, eat only half of your planned meal, then do something else for 20 minutes. Then come back, eat half of the remaining food, wait 20 minutes, and so on until you are finished eating. Remember, these are training exercises preparing you for the future. Tools you will be able to use. Don't go hungry now, just pledge to use the 20 minutes tool today at all meals so you can learn to do it.

Progress Focused Lying Posture Time

Block off 30 minutes during this day. Assume a lying posture, with a blanket and pillow positioned underneath your back, with you faceup. This exercise takes place somewhere quiet: in a private room, outside in the park under a tree, etc. For 20 or so minutes, you will observe your breath. Track it as you inhale, feel it as your rib cage and belly expand, listen as it makes its way out when you exhale. Imagine that the pure oxygen you bring in flows through your body, between the muscle fibers, to your toes, and through each chamber of your heart as it brings purity to your body. Know that each breath brings with it snow-white clarity and change. Each inflow makes its way through every area of your body, bringing with it the breeze of change, and each outflow means the exit of everything that has been holding you back. You've got the secret to transformation now. You've set it in motion with your exercise, and now you are directing your body to change, to adjust, to rid itself of toxins and sludge with each exhalation—to make you strong. For the final 10 minutes, focus on how much you have done. Focus on the change you have initiated and accumulated. Feel proud. Feel engaged. Feel happy.

Tofu Google

Take this day to google (or use your search engine of choice) tofu. Find a way to incorporate tofu into your life. Make a tofu recipe. Eat some tofu. The goal here is twofold: (1) to try tofu and get over the tofu hump, and (2) to introduce the exercise of making educated decisions regarding intake. Part of the barrier between "us and them" is lack of knowledge. This is an exercise in gaining a taste for soy-containing foods and getting used to expanding your horizons.

Playing Your Hand

Today, take 25 minutes to reflect on the "hand you have been dealt." Much of what has contributed to your failures so far has been trying to jump to end goals without the means to get there. Take an inventory today—on paper—of five personal strengths and weaknesses. Keep it in your wallet, purse, or smartphone. Think about how you will play your strengths and minimize your weaknesses. You have to make progress starting with what you have, and you don't want to waste time battling your weaknesses when you could be progressing.

For example, if one of your weaknesses is folding to sugar cravings late at night, list that. Then reflect on how you've decided not to put tons of weight on that point since it is a weakness. You won't take it on directly right away but rather leave it to wither by not paying attention to it, not worrying about it, and not letting it stop you from completing the program!

On the other hand, if one of your strengths is cooking or being organized or motivated, then list those. And consider how you will play to those strengths. Plan ahead a bit to make sure you eat recovery foods and have the tools to detox. Think about how you will capitalize on that motivation by working out and staying focused on the positive.

This important exercise will help you formulate a plan post catching point. No more blind sign-ups to diets. You are training to be deliberate in the future. Know thyself.

Recipe Planner Day

Use today to do the following things: (1) organize and review the recipes in this book, printing them and putting them somewhere if possible, and (2) take the time to pick one or two and plan a meal.

Specifically, decide which day you will make said meal and which day you will eat, realizing that you may need to make a meal and store it for later. It is not likely that you will be able to do this all today, unless it's your day off and you are looking for a project. The point here is to make this exercise doable. Get your arms around something that can actually be done by breaking it down into doable steps: identify a meal, identify a time and place to gather/buy ingredients, gather and buy the ingredients, plan the time for preparation, prepare the meal, store in a container or eat it.

Completing this task is important. Teach yourself that this type of meal preparation is not a "pie in the sky" but rather something you can do with some planning. Don't revolutionize your whole life at this point and try to make one of these every day—that won't work. Pick one or two. Get something done without exhausting yourself or dropping out. One thing at a time.

Look at the Wall

Enjoy your day today. Go to the mall. Watch some TV. Read a book. Take a swim.

Before you do, though, take 10 minutes (10 please, not 2 or 5) to reflect on what you have done. Really think about how you are in it now and—because you have come this far—*now you have something to lose*. You have banked some progress so when you do that next workout, whenever it may be, *you will* **not** *be starting at ground zero*. You have already changed a bit. Jumped a level. It is happening. Today, try not to think about where you are headed or where you want to be but rather how much you have accomplished so far. Realize that you are well into the race. You will never have to start over again because you already have put some work in.

Imagine that the next time you work out you are starting at a new level, a higher level than ever before. Think of your next workout as day 1—but beginning a new and higher-level program—one with a sweeter end point. Then imagine that when this program is over, you can have a day 1 at a new level, a higher level—any day 1 you want. You pick: CrossFit, hot yoga, insane home workouts, marathons, triathlons, whatever. It all starts with this new day 1 on this new level to which you have climbed. Great job. Feel glad for what you have done so far, and feel confident that the walls you've built won't let you go backward.

Here's another way to think of this: If you sacrificed to save $100—if you didn't go to the movies or didn't buy yourself medicine or went without new shoes to save $100—would you then blow that $100 on junk food? No way. You would be protective of it because you sacrificed to get it and would be loath to waste your sacrifice. You'd say, "Hold on! I worked hard to save that—don't just blow it!" Same thing here. Next time you work out, you're starting with $100 instead of nothing. Fantastic.

Post Workout Prep

Gather the following items today, five workouts in advance. Keep them with you either in your car, office, or home so that you have them the next five workouts.

Five Gatorade bottles of your flavor choice. For males I would recommend the 32 ounce and for females the 20 ounce.

Whey protein powder.

A funnel.

Have these items at the ready so that following your workout (within 45 minutes) you can drop one scoop of whey protein into the Gatorade,* mix, and drink.**

* You will need to pour out or drink about a third of the liquid to make room for the powder.

** Gatorade has realized the value of this mixture and is marketing a protein-Gatorade mix of its own, which is a suitable alternative.

Chromium Friday (or Wednesday, or Monday....)

Chromium day is the time to supplement or source chromium as an exercise in building your knowledge base and resources. That is, chromium is a potential tool for you to decrease sugar cravings in advance. Know which foods contain chromium and how it works (see chapter 9). Today, consume three servings of broccoli with black pepper and grape juice as a snack, meal, or premeal.

Sunrise Planning

Today make a plan to time one of your upcoming workouts for first thing in the day/morning. This is a great tool to have in your toolbox because it serves multiple purposes:

1. It gets the workout done. It is much easier to get through 30 minutes of exercise first thing in the morning as compared to after work/family/church/shopping/traffic/etc.

2. It provides for a fresh, good feeling all day. Multiple studies have shown that activity early in the day boosts metabolism and mood.

3. Most importantly, a workout performed after the fast of sleeping has no fuel from which to draw except fat. That is, although you are focused on recovery for the most part during this program, this is one time when you can't ignore that the body will exclusively burn fat.

So learn this lesson and bank it as a weapon against obesity going forward.

Throw Stuff Out

OK, now this one I know can be tough. If you aren't ready, swap this out for another recovery. If you feel OK, go into your pantry or refrigerator and throw out some junk food. Chips, candy bars, sugar cereal, etc.—the obvious stuff. Importantly, don't throw it *all* out! Remember, you are doing things in chunks, collecting little bits of progress. You are not interested in making huge, rash changes that will wreck your progress. Little things, little things, little things. Throw out one or two or three things. Learn the skill. You won't even notice. Enjoy the rest of the day; you are doing great.

Nonprocessed Island

Your body will love this detox. For one day, keep processed foods out of your system and undergo a natural cleanse of toxins. Not for a month, or a week—just one day.

How to do this? Anything that has been changed by man is off limits. Today is fruits, vegetables, healthy proteins (fish, beans [garbanzo, kidney, lima, black], ground turkey, baked chicken), whole-grain bread, steel-cut oats, brown rice, whole-grain cereal, soy milk, and just about anything labeled "organic." The one exception here will be peanut butter. Use peanut butter on whole-grain bread to fill up if you are still hungry (though still try to use an organic brand if possible).

Remember, you are arming yourself with tools for the future and reprogramming your body. This day will help you rid your body of years of toxin buildup (even cancer-causing agents) so that you feel fresh and strong. It will also teach you that you can look beyond processed foods to eat and survive.

If you were stranded on an island without processed foods, you would not die. You would switch to survival mode. Intake of food for life, just like gas for your car. One day. You can do it.

Flax Granola Snack Prep

Today's recovery is straightforward. Prepare two plastic containers containing three cups of flax granola and two containers filled with as many blueberries as you can eat. Store these for snacks or premeal options. Mix with yogurt to add taste. If you eat one today, make the replacement combination right away so that when you go to sleep tonight, there are two snacks prepared for the upcoming days. Planning is an important skill. Nice work.

Old Faithful

Eat every two to three hours today. This is a classic, and it is science supported. We talked a lot about the body defaulting to survival because we are made a certain way. This is the same thing—if you don't eat for five hours, the body will slow down the burn (and snuff your afterburn, as discussed in chapter 6). It is also true that at the two-hour mark, you won't be pushing old ladies down the stairs to get your pizza; you'll be under control and less likely to overeat. I stole this one from the standard diet plans, but hey—it's a tool that works.

Catching Anonymous

Today, work the principles of the "anonymous" groups—Overeaters, Alcoholics, etc. Admit that you are powerless alone over this struggle with weight loss and fitness, and trust in another power (in this case, the power of recovery and the catching point) to restore you to sanity. Turn your life over to that power. Submit to it, believe it, and trust it. Reflect on your newfound focus on the catching point and let every other distraction fall to the side, no matter how enticing it may seem. Commit to finish the program. Withhold judgement until you get to that point. Remind yourself that you'll never have to quit, that the program supports you when you are up and down and will carry you through to the finish. Smile and be happy. You've finally found a way out.

CHAPTER 10—

The Program

OK, HERE WE ARE. Here are the instructions for your catching point exercises. As you read these, keep in mind that ultimately you are after that addicting taste of success. You are aiming to hold on as long as you possibly can, at all costs and through an unlimited number of adjustments, to get to that catching point which will fuel your momentum. Every little thing you do toward the program counts. It all adds up toward your goal. Little things build on little things that build on little things to get you there.

The Workouts

1. Obey the rules at all times. These are nonnegotiable.

2. Check off as many tasks as possible in the 84 days. Check your score against the transformation grades. (More on this below.)

3. Repeat any task as desired. Listen to your body.

That's it. It is that simple. The key, of course, is that this program is adjustable and thereby un-quittable. And finishing. You care about finishing. Throughout this book, we have made the point over and over that you too can reach these fitness goals and make changes, that you have the same potential as anyone who has done it. We've stressed that it isn't endurance of pain and suffering that you need but a doable path. This program is doable. It is tailored to react and adjust to your feedback—to let up when you need it to, and to be there when you feel good. Use the principles in this book *to pace yourself.* Take 10 days off in a row if you need to, but *finish.* This is the only "must do" for the entire program, that you stay on it until you reach your goal.

In order to stay on course, use the adjustability function and use your options. Wipe out days that don't fit your feedback, and allow your program to recalibrate. Watch the tallies. At the end of the levels, you will have something in your toolbox (chapter 2)—meaning that you will have done work and contributed to your transformation. *It is up to you to see how fast you can get to that point.* You stay after it and get to the next level. Level 1, level 2, level 3, done. Chase it, love it, own that goal—make it your mission. Focus on that number and make it the center of your universe. Use the workout days to initiate recovery changes.

When you feel good, and ready, and fresh, and motivated, and on board—do the next workout. Some are harder than others. Do not feel restrained by any predetermined schedule, and do not feel restrained by the difficulty level. The essence of the first nine chapters is that the schedule absolutely, categorically *must* be flexible and dynamic in response to how you feel. It won't work any other way.

If you aren't "feeling" the scheduled workout, replace it with one that you *are* feeling. Simply switch to the option that fits your mood and let the program recalibrate. Pick a workout that you think you can do and want to do. Do it, then focus on recovery. If you feel great, and strong, and motivated, pull in another the next day, or pick one with a higher difficulty. The point is, do what you feel like doing. Don't force a square peg into a round hole. If you don't feel like working out at all on a certain day, replace the workout with a recovery, or a day off. *The program is based on years of research and collaboration to readjust according to your changes, track your progress, and keep you on target.* Trust it. Follow your gut. Wait for the change.

The program is tailored to get you to change by responding to your feedback. The same is true if you wake up on an "off day" feeling energetic and motivated. I want you to listen to the signals being put forth by your body and respond accordingly and *not* stick to the schedule as it is written. The order is meaningless—all you need to do is check off as many boxes as possible in 84 days. Look, you could do it again after 84 days and try to beat your original score!

Follow the cues explained in the earlier chapters. Embrace the motivation and energy when it presents itself, and respect the fatigue and shutdown when those feelings emerge. *In this way you will never be fighting your program but riding the momentum to the end.*

The recovery lines contain options as described in the book: from diet related (such as the vinegar vegetable, salmon, or soy bean product options) to active recovery (massage or foam rolling or the relaxation sequence) to mind-body complex interventions (prayer, meditation, nature walks, etc.). Intermix the recovery options with the workout options *according to how you feel.* Critical to your success will be listening to your body's signals so that you can maintain motivation for the entirety of the program and finish level 3. Each one of you is likely to have a different pattern in the end, according to the signals your body sends you. The important thing is to pick an option each day. Get to level 3. Remember, there is no quitting or restarting—if you feel like you want to chuck it, use some off-day options. Use 10 in a row if you want. Of course, you can do each option as many times as there is space in the right column of the table.

The Third Lap

After starting this program, at some point you undoubtedly will feel like quitting. During any significant undertaking, there will be a period of discouragement, which we can call "the third lap." A mile is four times around the track. If you set out to run a mile—a significant undertaking for most of us—you will be full of energy and motivation during the first lap, because it's new, you're excited, etc. The second lap gets you to halfway. You are driven to get to the halfway point because it means much of what you need to do is finished, so the remaining portion looks doable and you are psyched. The fourth lap is it! You're driving it home! You're really going to do it! But the third lap sucks totally. You aren't halfway, you aren't finishing, and you are really getting tired of this crap. It's during the third lap that you start to question why you started this at all, wondering what is the point. During the third lap of this program, you likely won't even want to look at or keep track of these stupid options!

Fine! Do nothing for as many days as it takes for your brain to start thinking about dieting and exercising again. *Then come back and check off some more boxes.* Check off a workout, stimulate recovery, use some recovery options, and so forth. The idea is to do as much as possible in the 84 days *without starting over!*

The 7/10 Rule

Remember the slowly moving cliff. When you start, you will be all fired up to get exercising. You may feel like this on day 2, you may not. If you do, work out again. If not, use recovery or nothing options in order to let the cliff move away and keep your motivation fire burning. Be very aware and careful of that fire. Do not stomp it out by overdoing it. Do not run off the cliff. You've got to keep motivated for 84 days. When you get through all 84 days, you will have made significant changes to your body—you will be different from the inside out. At that point, the sky is the limit.

One specific piece of advice as you embark on your journey: have more active days than not. This is where the 7/10 rule comes in. As you go along, responding each day to how you feel, how your schedule changes, and so on, keep in mind how many days you've used a workout or recovery options and how many days you've used a nothing option. Try to keep the "do something" options—workout or recovery—just a bit more than the do nothing options. Each 10 or so days, reflect and make sure that of those days, 6 or 7 were do somethings. Of course, crazy weeks come up, your mind tanks on you occasionally, you get a cold, whatever—but on average, try to have 7 good, do something days for every 10. Over the course of the program, having more active days will pace your progress and start to instill that momentum for a long-term lifestyle. In the long run, after you've left me and moved on to the fitness mainstream, you will see that successful people still eat ribs and ice cream on occasion, but in general they have more good days than not. So, it's a useful principle for the program and a great long-term habit.

Also, consider beating the system if you can. For example, use a recovery and workout option on the same day. Have a great workout and then do the relaxation sequence later in the day if you have time. If you do that, you can throw extra points in to increase your points to date and your progress. This is literally and figuratively going "outside the box," which I encourage.

The Magic Number Eight and the Random Day of Awesomeness

There is a secret about the eighth workout. My guess is that it is a secret because you have rarely reached the eighth workout, if ever. (Understandable. Please see the preceding nine chapters for an explanation as to why.) But now, given the flexibility, adjustability, and dynamic nature of this program, you can get to that eighth workout. The eighth workout is an internal catching point. That is, the entire program aims to translocate you from the current wrong side of the entry barrier to the catching point, as in figure 7, chapter 1. Once there, you will have what you have been looking for. It turns out, fortunately, that you will have a bit of a taste of your end product about one-quarter of the way through this program. Prior to workout 8, you will be trying like heck-water to keep motivated and on track. Once you get to workout 8, *even this program* will get easier. After eight workouts (not any amount of *time*, mind you, but eight *workouts*), you will start eyeing that extras option. You will start thinking about what you eat on your own. You will start looking forward to the next workout. You will start feeling it. Recognize that drive, that accelerant, as what you are after. It may wane for a day or two afterward, but you will be able to recapture it through recovery. As an added tool, keep your focus on crazy number eight as a short-term goal.

The random day of awesomeness will catch you totally off guard (hence the clever name). While you are thinking about recovery changes and swiping days and staying on board until the end, a workout day will come when you feel like you could turn over a car. You'll start exercising and feel like you've been energized beyond your wildest dreams, like you could work out for 10 hours. Go with it. Harness it. Crush it. Embrace that energy and do as much as you can. Remember, you are looking for totals at the end, so if one day you found a bunch of valuable stamps at discounted prices or a bunch of $100 bills scattered about your room, you would gather as much as possible. Do that here too. Then recover. Enjoy it.

Be dynamic. Be responsive. Be attentive. Don't restart. Complete 84 (or more) tasks, of which at least 40 are nothing. Transform yourself. Catch a new lifestyle. Smile. Buy some yoga pants and get ninja abs. You can do it. Really.

The Catching Point Transformation: 7 Core Rules for 12 weeks[28]

1. **No restart.** This is critical—*it's the most important rule.* Mark off the tasks as you make your way through, and keep track of the points. If you miss a day, or two, or a week, *do not start over.* On the day you are ready to return, begin where you left off. It is much better to get 30 things done (vs. the entire 84) in 12 weeks than to start over. As explained in the earlier chapters, it is a fundamental mistake to quit and start over, always aiming for perfect attendance. You will not have perfect attendance on this program. Get as much done as you can. *No restarts.*

2. **No quitting.** Once you are on, you are on for 84 days. Even if you don't do another thing after your first workout, your score is 1 at the end of 84 days. Of course, you won't do that; you will come back in after 10 or 12 days when you get the itch. It's like the old television mafia rule—once you are in you cannot get out.

3. **No sugary drinks during the 12 weeks**. Zero. This means no sodas, no sweet tea, no sports drinks, no fruit drinks—except as part of the post-workout protein glycogen replenishment recovery from Chapter 9. Lots of water, black coffee, and unsweetened tea or sugar-free soda. Even on off days. Just for the 12 weeks.

4. **No getting drunk.** Sorry. You can go out and celebrate your transformation later.

28 These stand for all 12 weeks, regardless of daily assignment. Stick to these the entire time. Intermittently reread these.

5. **Sleep at least 50 hours a week.** That is approximately 7 hours a day. Keep track. If somehow you have a 5-hour day, be deliberate about making it up as soon as possible. The body changes during sleep. You are working for change.

6. **Eat breakfast.** This is an "oldie but goodie" and it has stood the test of time. Keep your metabolism in high gear. Eat clean for change.

7. **Do not sit for more than 45 consecutive minutes.** If you have a desk job or any other tendency to sit for prolonged periods of time, deliberately break it up before the 1-hour mark (each hour) and go for a short walk, stretch, or engage in outright exercises. If you are sitting because of excessive screen time (smartphones, television, etc.), take note.

The Catching Point Transformation: 12-Week Transformation Task Point Table

Workouts	Points
Level 1 Walk = 3 points each	
Burpee Challenge = 3 points each	
Level 1 Alpha = 3 points each	
Level 1 Beta = 3 points each	
Level 1 Gamma = 3 points each	
Level 1 Delta = 3 points each	
Level 1 Epsilon = 3 points each	
Level 1 Zeta = 3 points each	
Level One Eta = 3 points each	
Level 1 Theta = 3 points each	
Level 1 Iota = 3 points each	
Level 2 Walk = 4 points each	
Level 2 Alpha = 4 points each	

Level 2 Beta = 4 points each	
Level 2 Gamma = 4 points each	
Level 2 Delta = 4 points each	
Level 2 Epsilon (Gym) = 5 points each	
Level 2 Zeta (Gym) = 5 points each	
Level 2 Eta (Gym) = 5 points each	
Level 2 Theta (Gym) = 5 points each	
Level 2 Iota (Gym) = 5 points each	
Level 3 Alpha = 6 points each	
Level 3 Beta = 6 points each	
Level 3 Gamma = 6 points each	
Level 3 Delta = 6 points each	
Level 3 Epsilon = 6 points each	
Recoveries	
Mediterranean Quinoa Salad = 1 point	
Catching Point Chili = 1 point	
Lettuce Wraps = 1 point	
Avocado Ranch Dressing = 1 point	
Asiago Chicken Sausage = 1 point	
Crispy Brazil Nut Bars = 1 point	
Egg Muffins = 1 point	
Catching Point Mega Salad = 1 point	
Lemon Pepper Green Beans and Almonds = 1 point	
Chicken Stir-Fry = 1 point	
Chicken Tortilla Soup = 1 point	
Baked Garlic Fries = 1 point	
The Sleeper = 1 point	
Soy Stew = 1 point	
Christmas Eve Baccalà = 1 point	
Soy Shake and a Nap = 1 point	
Selenium and Molybdenum = 1 point	
Leucine Trigger and Hot Tub = 1 point	
Raw Vegetables and Fruit = 1 point	
Water and Vinegar = 1 point	
Focused Imagery = 1 point	
The Relaxation Sequence = 2 points	

Massage, Active Release, and/or Myofascial Release = 2 points	
Lunasin and Soluble Fiber Cleanse = 1 point	
The Snack Planner = 2 points	
Recon = 2 points	
20 Minutes = 1 point	
Progressive Focused Lying Posture = 1 point	
Tofu Google = 1 point	
Playing Your Hand = 2 points	
Look at the Wall = 1 point each	
Post-Workout Prep = 1 point	
Chromium Day = 1 point	
Sunrise Planning = 2 points	
Throw Stuff Out = 2 points	
Nonprocessed Island = 2 points	
Flax Granola Snack Prep = 1 point	
Old Faithful = 1 point	
Catching Anonymous = 2 points	
Off Days = 0.5 point each	

Points	Translation
165	Perfect score. Let's see who can do this.
100–164	Exceptional. Top 5%. Proceed to any program or activity you wish. Enjoy your new life.
70–100	Superb. Top 15%. Proceed to midlevel mainstream transitional program before moving into unlimited space.
40–70	Excellent. Consider repeating the catching point program before transitioning to outside program. Aim for higher score.
< 40	Nice. You will do great with one more time through. Getting the hang of it.

Below is a sample of what your program might look like when you finish. Each time you complete a task, write the corresponding point value in the right column. At the end of the 12 weeks, simply add up all your scores and see where you land on the table. In this example, the person ended with a 92—a superb score. This person is encouraged to move on to a mainstream program of their choice, knowing that it will be so much easier now that they're on the other side of the catching point. If you don't like your score, take another 12-week challenge. (Remember, don't ever start over!)

Sample Program

Workouts	Points
Level 1 Walk = 3 point each	3, 3, 3, 3, 3
Burpee Challenge = 3 points each	
Level 1 Alpha = 3 points each	3
Level 1 Beta = 3 points each	3, 3
Level 1 Gamma = 3 points each	3
Level 1 Delta = 3 points each	3
Level 1 Epsilon = 3 points each	3, 3
Level 1 Zeta = 3 points each	3
Level 1 Eta = 3 points each	3
Level 1 Theta = 3 points each	3, 3
Level 1 Iota = 3 points each	
Level 2 Walk = 4 points each	4, 4, 4
Level 2 Alpha = 4 points each	4
Level 2 Beta = 4 points each	
Level 2 Gamma = 4 points each	4
Level 2 Delta = 4 points each	
Level 2 Epsilon (Gym) = 5 points each	
Level 2 Zeta (Gym) = 5 points each	
Level 2 Eta (Gym) = 5 points each	
Level 2 Theta (Gym) = 5 points each	
Level 2 Iota (Gym) = 5 points each	

Level 3 Alpha = 6 points each	
Level 3 Beta = 6 points each	
Level 3 Gamma = 6 points each	
Level 3 Delta = 6 points each	
Level 3 Epsilon = 6 points each	
Recoveries	
Mediterranean Quinoa Salad = 1 point	1
Catching Point Chili = 1 point	1, 1
Lettuce Wraps = 1 point	
Avocado Ranch Dressing = 1 point	
Asiago Chicken Sausage = 1 point	1
Crispy Brazil Nut Bars = 1 point	
Egg Muffins = 1 point	
Catching Point Mega Salad = 1 point	1, 1
Lemon Pepper Green Beans and Almonds = 1 point	
Chicken Stir-Fry = 1 point	
Chicken Tortilla Soup = 1 point	1
Baked Garlic Fries = 1 point	
The Sleeper = 1 point	
Soy Stew = 1 point	
Christmas Eve Baccalà = 1 point	
Soy Shake and a Nap = 1 point	
Selenium and Molybdenum = 1 point	1, 1
Leucine Trigger and Hot Tub = 1 point	1
Raw Vegetables and Fruit = 1 point	1, 1, 1
Water and Vinegar = 1 point	
Focused Imagery = 1 point	1
The Relaxation Sequence = 2 points	
Massage, Active Release, and/or Myofascial Release = 2 points	2
Lunasin and Soluble Fiber Cleanse = 1 point	1
The Snack Planner = 2 points	
Recon = 2 points	2
20 Minutes = 1 point	1, 1
Progressive Focused Lying Posture = 1 point	
Tofu Google = 1 point	1
Playing Your Hand = 2 points	

Look at the Wall = 1 point each	
Post-Workout Prep = 1 point	
Chromium Day = 1 point	
Sunrise Planning = 2 points	2
Throw Stuff Out = 2 points	
Nonprocessed Island = 2 points	
Flax Granola Snack Prep = 1 point	
Old Faithful = 1 point	
Catching Anonymous = 2 points	
Off Days = 0.5 point each	0.5, 0.5, 0.5, 0.5, 0.5, 0.5, 0.5, 0.5, 0.5, 0.5, 0.5, 0.5, 0.5, 0.5, 0.5, 0.5, 0.5, 0.5, 0.5, 0.5, 0.5, 0.5, 0.5, 0.5, 0.5, 0.5, 0.5, 0.5, 0.5, 0.5, 0.5, 0.5, 0.5, 0.5, 0.5, 0.5, 0.5, 0.5, 0.5, 0.5, 0.5, 0.5
Total	92

Points	Translation
165	Perfect score. Let's see who can do this.
100–164	Exceptional. Top 5%. Proceed to any program or activity you wish. Enjoy your new life.
70–100 **(92)**	Superb. Top 15% Proceed to midlevel mainstream transitional program before moving into unlimited space.
40–70	Excellent. Consider repeating the catching point program before transitioning to outside program. Aim for higher score.
< 40	Nice. You will do great with one more time through. Getting the hang of it.

There is a simpler way to translate your goal. The actual catching point is a number—a number that reflects an exercise capacity. This critical point represents the transition point beyond which healthy living is fun and easy and the crushing unpleasantries of the diet cycle drop off (figure 20). The biological resistance that mounts against a human being when they abruptly restrict their calories and superimpose exercise stress gradually decreases as the exercise capacity (defined in units called Met-Minutes) increases. Importantly, it drops precipitously beyond 210 Met-Minutes (the X in figure 20), making things much, much easier.

A few important things to know about this. First, 210 Met-Minutes can be roughly translated to activity—approximately the ability to jog for 30 minutes without stopping, or slowly bike for an hour, or swim laps for 40 minutes, and so on. This capacity point can be used (very roughly now, don't get too carried away) as a surrogate for the catching point.[29] So, if you are not in the mood to add up points and find where you fall on the translation table, you can instead work toward this capacity point.

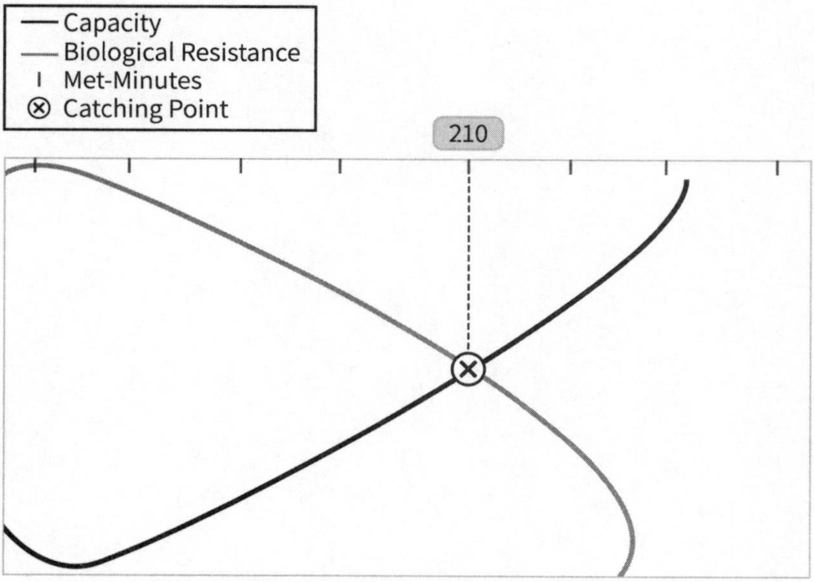

Capacity vs. Biological Resistance to Weight Loss, as defined by Met-Minutes

Figure 20. The catching point curve.

Second, if you remember the pool-to-tools analogy from chapter 2, the inability to execute 210 Met-Minutes leaves you at a permanent disadvantage (beyond the point of this book, which is that you will always have suffocating resistance) when trying to change because you could try

29 These numbers may vary a bit. Remember, everyone is different (chapter 2).

to follow an exercise program until the cows come home and you will never impact change by burning calories.

Third, exercise alters food preferences. So, the combination of quieting resistance, acquiring effective tools for calorie burning, and altering food preferences toward healthy choices results in a rather abrupt change, beyond which all of this is easy.

PART 3:

Beyond Fitness

CHAPTER 11—

The Catching Point at Work and Throughout Life

"You can't deliver mail!"

"Why not?"

"I guess you're right. It's just walking around putting it into boxes."

—*Seinfeld,* Season 8, Episode 10

I HESITATED TO INCLUDE THIS chapter because it really simplifies the book, kind of taking away from the brilliant doctor's eloquently constructed plan. But let's face it: all you have to do is stay engaged. You just have to be there. Physically be on board the whole time. That's really all it is. I don't want you to quit, because in the long run the lifestyle will catch for you—and that is what changes your life.[197] Consider a real-life example, then some applications beyond fitness.

My Story

Because this book and this program are a personal effort (rather than some ghostwritten nonsense intended to exploit the struggles of overweight people, which, in my opinion, is not much different than making money by selling magic sugar pills to desperate dying cancer patients, but let's not go down that rabbit hole right now), I thought it would be appropriate to share my own experience with the catching point principles.

Importantly, I was very much "into fitness" for the early part of my life, until about age 24. I stood very much amongst the smiley in-shape people as one of them, passing judgment on the weak and feeling superior because the fatties were either too dumb or too uncool to overcome. I condescended and patronized my own loved ones because of their apparent lack of knowledge or willpower. I watched them start diet after diet and exercise program after exercise program, only to fail a few days in. "You gotta really want it," I told them.

I stood very much amongst the smiley in-shape people as one of them, passing judgment on the weak and feeling superior because the fatties were either too dumb or too uncool to overcome.

Now, fast-forward 10 years, and I'm terribly overweight and out of shape after a decade of drinking, smoking, eating fast food, and not sleeping well. I got my act together, finished my training, had some kids, and went to work. I was still overweight and unhealthy, but fixing that was on my list of things to do. In fact, I developed this routine when I traveled. I would enter the airport bookstore, buy two bodybuilding magazines and usually one fitness book, and read on the plane about programs for "abs transformation" or "how to get shredded in eight weeks." The allure was fantastic! I loved bodybuilding, the idea of being ripped and having abs, and could certainly do *anything* for eight weeks—especially if it meant looking like that!

Of course I never did it. But wait. On one particular trip I found a book that contained running schedules for beginners who wanted to run a marathon. Great! Fantastic! Finally this would be doable because I would be able to run in the morning before work instead of trying to find time to drive to the gym for those other programs, shop for the chicken, etc. Here I could just follow the directions, run a marathon, and *then* I'd be good for starting that ripped program because I'd be "cleansed." And what was so great was I wouldn't have to think too much—this thing literally said, Monday do this, Tuesday do this, and so on. Perfect.

> "Shit, this is hard. Like impossible. No wonder people can't get back over this hump."

I must have spent $10,000 on diet books and programs and online subscriptions over the years. I was in shape before, even a real athlete, but just couldn't find my way back. Sound familiar? So here is where you may expect the story to go, "Then *one day*, I blah blah blah after I had a heart attack or my Uncle Butch got diabetes or I had to walk upstairs because the elevator broke." Nope. None of that stuff happened to me. I was busy with kids and my job, so I just didn't do it. Somehow getting in shape kept falling off that list of things to do. I figured I'd get to it one day when everything else slowed down. Meanwhile, I remained feeling starved and pissed and tired.

What did happen during this time, though, was that a new thought emerged deep inside my brain which, prior to this point on my life, I would have never considered: "Shit, this is hard. Like impossible. No wonder people can't get back over this hump." And with that thought, all of the times I assumed exercise and diet experiences were the same for everyone came crashing to the forefront of my mind. The times I would drone on about how "all you have to do" is this and that and you will be in shape like me were replayed, and the realization set in that I (and 99 percent of trainers and authors and infomercial stars) were just describing *what we did* and that it *didn't apply* to these poor people. They were in a different place, in need of a whole different set of instructions and advice—and then on top of that, *each one of them* was an individual. And now I was with them, unable to cross back over. So for the next 10 years I studied this phenomenon, this amazing expanse between the haves and the have-nots and the fantasy bridges from one side to the other.

Then I put it to the test. I didn't announce to anyone that I was starting anything. I didn't declare a "day 1." I didn't set a goal, I didn't make a schedule. I didn't restrict my eating. Instead I looked at my children and silently decided to "put some money in the bank" for them when I got the chance. Instead of going the rest of my life without ever exercising because I couldn't stay on any of those programs, I just resolved to stay fat (it was clear I could not change that) but get in some jogs once in a while so my heart would have some jolts and maybe shake off some of the grease it must have been sitting in.[30] This experience was comparable to, say, volunteering at a soup kitchen one day. Most people aren't looking to transform their lives when they volunteer; they just want to do something good on that day and feel warm and cozy about themselves when they go to bed that night. Most people aren't looking to quit their jobs and run a charity when they volunteer. Similarly, when I ran around the block, I wasn't doing it as part of a grand master plan to get ripped. It was just that one time so when I went to bed I could feel glad about something I did during the day.

I felt sore and couldn't sleep right after those jogs. But when I sat down to watch TV and eat ice cream on the days that I had run, I felt stupendous. And it was fun. I wasn't under any pressure to meet deadlines, keep a schedule, or starve. I *added* good feelings to my day by jogging a bit (actually they were more like walk a little, jog a little, walk a little, done) with no restrictions. I got some fresh air and breathed heavy for a bit. When I went to bed on those days, I felt like I had done something good. Felt like maybe I volunteered for an hour, helped someone who was struggling find a meal, or lent a hand to a junior coworker that day.

Then a magical (that's right, magical) force oozed into my life. I started to *want* to run. I started to look forward to it. I started to make time for it because it was something I *wanted* to do—and it had nothing to do with losing weight, eating less, or following a schedule. I had an itty-bitty feeling of accomplishment at the end of the days I jogged, and I felt good about it. I created a positive link between exercise and my brain, so my brain—in its infinite complexity and wisdom—said OK, since that gives us good feelings, let's do it more.

Admittedly, at this point my efforts were purposeful. I was trying to create that positive link because I felt like it was the wormhole through which people could crawl to get back in shape and accomplish their fitness goals. I wanted it to work. And it did. My body got stronger, and my ability to run farther and faster slowly improved. It then became a game. When I sat down on Friday night to relax, I would reflect on how many miles I had run that week. The more the better. So the next week I would run when I could, when I had time, *when I felt like it.* Over time I felt better and better, and every night I ate ice cream or cookies.

30 Importantly, I was not doing this to live longer, get in shape, be skinny, or engage in any other "goal-oriented" behavior.

But sure enough, even knowing all the things written above in this book, you can overdo it while pursuing those good feelings. If you overdo it, run ahead of the moving cliff, you can get some negative feedback, then push through it in search of that great, warm, cozy feeling at the end of the day with miles under your belt. When that would happen to me, my mind would literally change. Literally I would have thoughts like, "You only live once, kid. Why mess around with all this running and crap?" What?! For 10 years and just last week I've wanted to feel better, look better, and so on. Where did this thought come from? *It came from the implementation of a goal and schedule* (the weekly mile tracking). My focus went to that and off my biofeedback mechanisms. I stopped listening to my body and started chasing a number.

So I would lay off, rest a few days, then come back—because I understood this principle and recognized that thought as an indicator that I was off the cliff. But still I wanted to do more. Run farther, get stronger. So I started doing push-ups during the walks. Then I started looking for stairs to run up. The more I did out there, the better I felt during the week—as long as I didn't overdo it and go off the cliff. And I had all the time in the world, because really what I was doing was nothing, right? I wasn't officially trying to do anything but feel good about myself on a day-by-day basis, so there were no deadlines.

Gradually, the decisions I made when I wasn't running started to depend on running. That is, I would defer a beer here and there because I wanted to run the next day. I started drinking Gatorade and protein after the runs so my body would get stronger for the next one. I was going to bed earlier because I wanted my body to rebuild stronger during sleep. I took vitamins and protein supplements before bed. Of note, and at the risk of being ridiculously repetitive, none of this had anything to do with weight or fat loss. I was simply feeling proud about my progress with running. It was catching.

As I was driving one day, I was daydreaming about martial arts. I mean, doesn't every boy/man at some point wish he would have done martial arts? Don't we all wish on some level that we were black belts in something or ninjas, or at least a little more Bruce Lee-like? I wondered, since I had been running, if I could tolerate a martial arts class. I figured I could really feel good about myself then.[31]

---

31 It is worth noting that had I started eating boiled rice and drinking spring water at this point in an attempt to be really awesome, it would have all crashed and burned.

Long story short, I found a gym with tons of classes offering plenty of times for me to attend when available. After going a few times, the same sort of "good feelings" followed, and I got a look at real fighters. At this point in my life, though, a very important realization had already set in for me—one that I am trying to convey to you, my beloved readers—and that is: *the road to failure for me would have been to start following their training and diet programs to the letter in an attempt to join them at their level.*

Business types call this an entry barrier. Lots of people have lots of good ideas all the time. Why aren't entrepreneurial millionaires being spawned every day, then? In my particular field, people think of great ideas for medical devices or drugs every five minutes, but rarely does an individual found a company and grow to any significant sales success. On the other hand, when Pfizer brings an erection pill to market, they make 50 go-zillion dollars. Could I have done that? Even if I'd thought of it (which I didn't, for full disclosure)? No! The reason is the entry barrier is too high. These companies have knowledge of things like market analysis, manufacturing ramp-up, supply chains, and on and on—stuff I have no idea about. I would have to learn these things, find funding to make most of it happen, then find time to orchestrate the whole thing. I would have *to get to the same starting point* as an established company before I could actually have a chance to market and sell my erection pill. I would have to overcome that entry barrier. Hence all the people walking around declaring, "OMG, I thought of that 10 years ago!" when something new comes out. Yeah, you did—but you didn't have the means to translate your idea to reality.

Now, back to my story. The difference between those real fighters and me comprised an entry barrier. When they showed up to work out, they were operating from a different level. If I wanted to be like them, I had a few years of base-work to do before I could train six days a week and eat clean as a whistle, just as it would take a few years of work to establish a supply chain, ramp up manufacturing, and define market segments for my medical device. I couldn't just ask one of these fighters for their program so I could start it on Monday and in eight weeks compete in a UFC fight. That would be stupid.

I needed to learn the rules, learn the components of the sport, and learn basic defense so I didn't get knocked out in the first minute. With my focus on these things, and not on those guys who were already competitive, I could get some small satisfactions and feel happy about the whole thing, but more importantly, the eating and exercise parts were silently beginning to "catch."[32] They were becoming things that I wanted to do. My brain started to look at working out and eating clean as fun instead of a drag list of things that had to be done so I could look pretty.

At this point I was home free. I had crossed back over. I was having fun, was proud of my progress, and woke up each day driven by that kinetic force. Nothing breeds success like a little success.[33] After this point I started to follow traditional programs (CrossFit, battle strength training, etc.). I didn't change my diet too much, but I was burning so many calories that I started to slim down, and—you guessed it—that fueled a spark in me to eat a little better, and eventually I got into pretty good shape. The same thing can be seen throughout life in non-fitness-related situations as well. Let us consider a few.

Alcoholics Anonymous

Perhaps the most powerful example of the catching point principles outside of the fitness arena is Alcoholics Anonymous (AA). The AA system has been working for almost 80 years. It has had millions and millions of members, has no leadership, enjoys a worldwide presence, and consistently reports success rates.[198, 199] It doesn't involve medication, doesn't cost money, doesn't implement a schedule, has no forced accountability (it's anonymous!), and requires nothing of its members. Thousands of scientific papers have been written investigating the mechanisms of effect. Doctors and scientists are enamored with how exactly something like this can be effective and persist. Paper after paper has sought to discredit AA without success.

So how do they do it? They have a saying in AA: "Keep coming back."

AA meetings occur in many different settings, from upper middle class to impoverished neighborhoods. The scene is strikingly reproducible (and strikingly similar to weight-loss endeavors). New members stand up and tell stories of how their lives were ravaged by alcohol—lost their wives, kids, jobs, went to jail, and on and on. Nevertheless they can't fig-

32 Presumably by this point in the book, you are making these connections on your own. But if not, the key here for me was just adding things on. So far in this riveting story, I haven't "taken away" anything. No food restrictions, no freedom loss. Just doing positive things and—incidentally, accidentally, almost as a bonus—transforming on the inside along the way.

33 To be clear, this journey wasn't an accident. Through a unique combination of experiences—including medical school, residency, interventional radiology practice, sports, obese friends and relatives, formal nutritional training, and extensive exercise science research—this theory of a huge, largely invisible entry barrier evolved. I happened to be in a position to serve as a guinea pig for the strategy to overcome this situation, so I did, but I wouldn't ask you to try something if it was just some lucky road I stumbled upon or some accidentally discovered treasure that I really didn't understand. Just saying.

ure out how to quit. Despite incredible losses, they seem to find their way back to drinking. The others in the room nod in understanding, knowing exactly how this guy or girl feels and what they are going through because they have all been there.

But now they've changed. Sobriety has "caught" for them, and they aren't even interested in drinking anymore. How can someone make such a drastic transition? How can they resist the urge to drink? The new ones beg through tears for the answer. "Please help me," they say to the members. "Please tell me what to do!"

These alcoholics are very similar to the repeat failures of diets. They haven't reached that turning point, that "catch point" when their urge to drink subsides. So they ask for the secret. They ask for a pill. They look for a guide to tell them what to do to extinguish that feeling and help them transition to this other lifestyle. This lifestyle that seems so easy for those who live it. Is this sounding familiar? *It is easy for those who live it.* They don't feel that screaming, overwhelming, knee-buckling urge to drink (or eat, or quit diets) anymore because they've passed through that catching point. And how did they do it? Ask anyone who was successful and they will tell you the same thing. "Nothing to do, my friend—just keep coming back."[34]

There is no specific day to come or number of times to show up. Attend an AA meeting once a week, five times a day, or monthly—depending on how you feel. Just don't go back to ground zero. Instead, come back to a meeting.

The catching point diet is the same thing. You don't have to work out on Monday, Wednesday, and Friday, or even Monday and Friday. Just don't go back to ground zero. Come back to the workouts without starting over and you are headed for that magical catch point. (See, I'm not making this stuff up—it's out there.)

Moving

What about moving? Not move like wave your arms but move in the relocation sense. For most people, moving can be as stressful as a death, so how do we do it? It's like a forced implementation of the catching point principles. If your friend is having reservations after moving to a new

34 The other great way this organization articulates this point is by telling new members who want to know how many days until effect, "Stay until the miracle happens."

home, what kinds of things would you say? "Just give it time." "After a while this new place will feel just like home." "In time, you will adjust to this place just like you did when you lived in Wherever Town." And guess what? You'd be right.

Over time people do adjust. But not because they start living that way on day 1. Or don't take breaks. Or force themselves to meet an "adjustment deadline." They are stuck there, so they just live. They wake up each day and they stay in the new place, and over time, it catches. These same people will tell you years later that at some point the tide turned (their catching point, of course) and they started to know the streets, make some friends, find the grocery stores, etc., and they integrated to their new location almost without noticing it was happening. You have to just be there. Literally, in order to get something to "catch," you just have to continue to physically be wherever it is that that thing happens. This is not some idea I had on the way to work; this is a literal truth that plays itself out in life over and over. You may not notice it but it's right there, so common a principle that it escapes our direct attention.

Importantly, it doesn't really matter what the moved human does on day 1 or day 7. They could go to a garden club on day 1 and a pool party on day 7, or they could just watch TV and get gas on day 1 and begrudgingly go to work on day 7. Either way, it's the fact that they are stuck there over time that ultimately allows them to make that transition. Now, if they drove back to their old house and sat on the lawn on day 2 or 3—*that* would block their progress. Same thing here. If you just stay engaged for the 84 days, even if you think you aren't getting anything accomplished, I promise you are. Physically, mentally, and spiritually you are adapting to the new lifestyle just like people who move and become part of a new town and a new way of life over time. You are integrating with the in-shape people so that in the long run, you will quietly live amongst them and carry memories of this place in the back of your mind. But if you quit, go back to your old house, and sit on the lawn—declaring that you will just move another day—then you get stuck. So stay engaged.

God

I've got one more for you, and it's a doozy. How many people have you spoken with about religion? How many times have you heard the conversation between the analyst and the believer? For the analyst, religion has never "caught," so he or she wants an up-front explanation. Just as the active alcoholic or the repeat failure of diets wants a step-by-step guide to the other side, so does the analyzer of religion. But, at the risk of brutal repetition, lifestyle changes like that aren't realized through a set of instructions. You will never be able to explain to the analyst how you know what you know about God, or articulate to the alcoholic why you don't have to drink. Likewise the in-shape people can't explain to you why they don't struggle with fitness. *It is something that happens over time, and it happens because they are there.* It hasn't happened to you yet because you jump ship. These things "catch" when you aren't looking because you keep coming back. Very few people have shown up at church for the first time and left a believer. They kept coming back (usually for some other reason, like a spouse, or sickness, or hardship) and then unbeknownst to them, it became part of their life—and once that happened they had a foundation to work from and it became effortless.

The same thing will happen through this program for fitness. Just hang around it. Don't force it. Forget the predetermined plan. Make it part of your life. It will gather momentum on its own.

Money and Marriage

In chapter 2, we said that you can't make $10 million just by reading a book entitled *How to Make $10 Million*. That is true—however, working toward financial security from ground zero is a pure example of the catching point principle and is a direct parallel analogy to weight loss. If you start a program that says, "Save $10 a day every day for a year," you will run to the bank the first day and put in your $10. Maybe even the second and third. Eventually, though, your motivation for saving will wane and you won't feel like going to the bank anymore. The key to your success will be what you decide to do with the money that has already been deposited, just as the key to your fitness is deciding what you will do with the changes that follow from your first few workouts. If you protect those changes and hold on to them until you feel like working out again, then you will be on your way. If you quit and start over, you will never realize those changes. Same thing here. If you protect that first $20 or $30, when you come back you will be on your way and the next deposit will get you to $40—instead of starting over at zero. Even if you don't deposit for a month, when you go back you'll be at $50. At some point you will deposit enough money *that you won't want to quit*. You'll have enough that the thought of going back to zero would sicken you. In fact, you will begin to focus on your money in the bank because you're excited about it. That amount of money that changes things from a job to fun lies square on the catching point. Get yourself there and harness the momentum. But do it on your own schedule, as you can. As long as you don't go backward, you'll get there.

Consider the catching point transformation program as it applies to marriage. As we all know, more than half of all marriages end in divorce, nearly as miserable as the statistics for success with dieting. No doubt this is a complex issue, but let's just say for fun that we used the catching point program for our marriage. We sit down with our spouse or partner, and we lay out the next 84 days with 40 dates, 40 positive inputs (flowers, compliments, sincere recognition of something good, serving some beers to our game-watching guy), and 40 nothings. The schedule is set. Of course we won't be able to keep this schedule because of our jobs, kids, in-laws, etc., plus we are going to have days when we just don't feel like it.

Now, my guess is that the divorcées and chronically unhappy treat the program as we used to treat dieting. They get to day 3 when they owe their spouse some positive energy but they are so crabby they just cannot do it. So they chuck the whole thing and never come back to it or schedule a new start day some time down the road when they are feeling bad and concerned about it again. As a result they *never* get any of the 80 good things done and they make no progress.

What if they focused on getting as many of the 80 good things in as possible? What if we offered $50,000 if they could reach, say, 45 positive things by the end of the 84 days? What if they kept the focus on *not quitting* the whole program after day 3 but instead swiped it out and came back to the program because the 84 days wasn't over and they could still get the $50K? Do you think that couples at the end of those 84 days with 20 dates and 20 positive inputs to each other would be any farther along or better off than the couples who did nothing? Hmmmmm...just saying.

The Pursuit of Happiness

A piece of the puzzle on how to do this—be it for abstinence, peace, financial security, or weight loss—is to find joy in the process. Of course, you hate the process now because it's uncomfortable, you're hungry, you're irritable, and so on. But, the first 10 chapters of this book have outlined how to *not* feel like that. So, let's look at it another way now.

My wife hated running. Hated it. Said it made her itchy and hot and it was overall just no fun. And so it went for years and years *until* her father got lymphoma. At some point after his diagnosis my wife stumbled upon Team In Training, which, of all things, was an organization that sponsored running in support of lymphoma. She went for the first meeting because she wanted to support her dad (much like the ex-analyst who first went to church because his wife died or the alcoholic who went to AA because of a court order). Then she went to the first run for the same reason. Then she missed a few because she was sad and came down with a cold. Now—and here is the critical point—she went back to run five or six because she wanted to be part of the group. She wanted to be around these people who were united through lymphoma. She just wanted to be around them.

I am sure you can see where this is going. To this day my wife runs and runs. It "got on her" while she was hanging around running for a different reason, while *she was focused on the process, not the end* (see mindfulness discussion, chapter 9). She found solace in the process and got to the end. This, after starting and stopping at least 50 different running programs designed to train beginners for marathons. For those, her eyes were on the end product—a marathon or half marathon or whatever. For Team In Training she found joy in the process.

So for catching point members, be glad that you've immersed yourself in this. Feel good about any vegetable you eat or workout you are recovering from. Enjoy the relaxation sequence. Sleep well. Be proud of yourself because you are a part of something, you are involved in this program. And, since you can't quit, you will be for a few months. There are no predetermined workout days, so you won't get kicked out for not keeping some insane schedule. Even the days you do nothing you're a part of this family.

The Well of Positivity

Another consideration regarding the process is that the catching point program can be viewed as a well full of positive change options for your life. For the 84 days, go to the well each day and draw out something good to *add* to your life. You want to effect changes in your body by adding in things—by adding peace and recovery and cleansing strategies into your life, all things that will make you feel better. As the program progresses, imagine that you have been given a well full of positive options to draw from. Instead of struggling, fighting, resisting, etc., imagine in the morning that you'll walk out and *add in* something positive to your life. These things will help your day-to-day time during the program be pleasant, rewarding, and tranquil and serve as an alternative focus to the ends. That is, your satisfaction with the program (and with life and your change) will come from knowing that each day you've added in a little good. As a result, your capacity will increase over time and your chances of completing the program will remain high. Good for you. You're doing great. Stay with us.

CHAPTER 12—

Procedures, Drugs, and Behavioral Interventions

AT SOME POINT YEARS AGO, amidst all the clatter produced by fitness gurus and diet trainers, a surgeon wondered, "What if we just made the stomach smaller? Wouldn't that lead to weight loss?" And in fact it did. Patients collectively lost thousands of pounds. Diseases like diabetes and high blood pressure were stopped in their tracks, and even reversed.

But it was more than that. Years of research that followed uncovered treasures of unexpected hormones and hunger switches responsible for obesity, diabetes, heart disease, sleep apnea, and more, and a brand-new paradigm for weight loss was born. *The age-old custom of shaming folks for their lack of willpower had been debunked. There was clearly more to this than "no pain, no gain."*

Although the mechanisms responsible for weight loss following surgery turned out to be unrelated to early proposed mechanisms, the surgeries still worked. And it works even better now. Weight-loss surgery, now called "metabolic surgery," works by altering all four of the components of resistance described in part 1.

Importantly, none of these are "willpower implantation" procedures.

There are four basic categories of interventions: bypass surgeries (gastric bypass, Roux-en-Y), restrictive surgeries (lap bands, sleeve gastrectomy), endoscopic procedures (intragastric balloons, duodenal sleeves), and minimally invasive interventional radiology procedures (bariatric artery embolization, cryovagotomy). Importantly, none of these are "willpower implantation" procedures. They are ways to interrupt the body's survival-based resistance to dieting.

Regarding the last of these (and the most recently developed), interventional radiologists have generated ways to modify the resistance put forth by the body in the setting of dieting and exercise using very specific, nonsurgical, image-guided targeting techniques. A procedure called bariatric artery embolization involves accessing the artery in your groin or wrist (very much like a heart catheterization) and steering a small plastic catheter under X-ray guidance to the vessels that supply your stomach.[4] Small particles are then deployed to block the vessels supplying the portion of your stomach that produces—you guessed it!—ghrelin. By blocking these vessels, the hunger hormone ghrelin can be reduced, and patients are less hungry.

A second interventional radiology procedure developed for the management of body backlash involves freezing the nerve that carries the hunger signal from an empty stomach to the brain (the CATCH procedure [CryoAblation To Curb Hunger]). The underlying idea here again is to quiet the body's response to calorie restriction, thereby overcoming a piece of the backlash that causes people to fail. During this procedure, a needle is guided (with CT guidance) through the skin of the back toward the top of the stomach. A small ice zone is created with that needle, and the signals in the hunger nerve (technically called the vagus nerve) are shut down. A study done in 2019 showed that freezing that nerve reduced appetite at nearly every checkpoint after the procedure for at least six months.[200] Further, research in many different species, including human beings, has demonstrated that interruption of that nerve results in decreased appetite, weight loss, and/or interruption of weight gain.[201–203] Using interventional radiology to target the vagus nerve is a recent development that allows doctors to slow hunger signaling without surgery or implants – just a 20 minute needle procedure.

The first patient who underwent a cryovagotomy in the world (Melissa) gave us permission to share her journey. I include it because it illustrates the purpose of the procedure, which is to ease the transition to weight loss by doing something to the body, thereby continuing to debunk the idea that being overweight is a mental fortitude issue. By blocking hunger, patients may tolerate lifestyle changes easier. Limited numbers of cryovagotomy procedures have been performed at the time of this book's publication (a few other participants are pictured with their permission), but the point remains the same—changes made to the body will change the mind, ease your experience, and change your life (remember chapter 3). Conquering this issue using "mind over matter" is a wild goose chase. The same body changes can be made using the program outlined in this book. That said, the combination of any two may be the most powerful tool(s) we have to date.

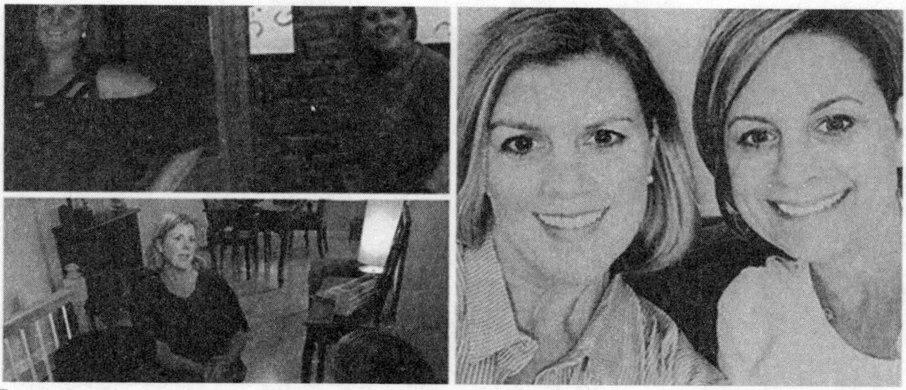

The very first cryovagotomy patient, Melissa. Images from the early years following the procedure demonstrating Melissa's progressive weight loss (left). Melissa four years after her procedure (right).

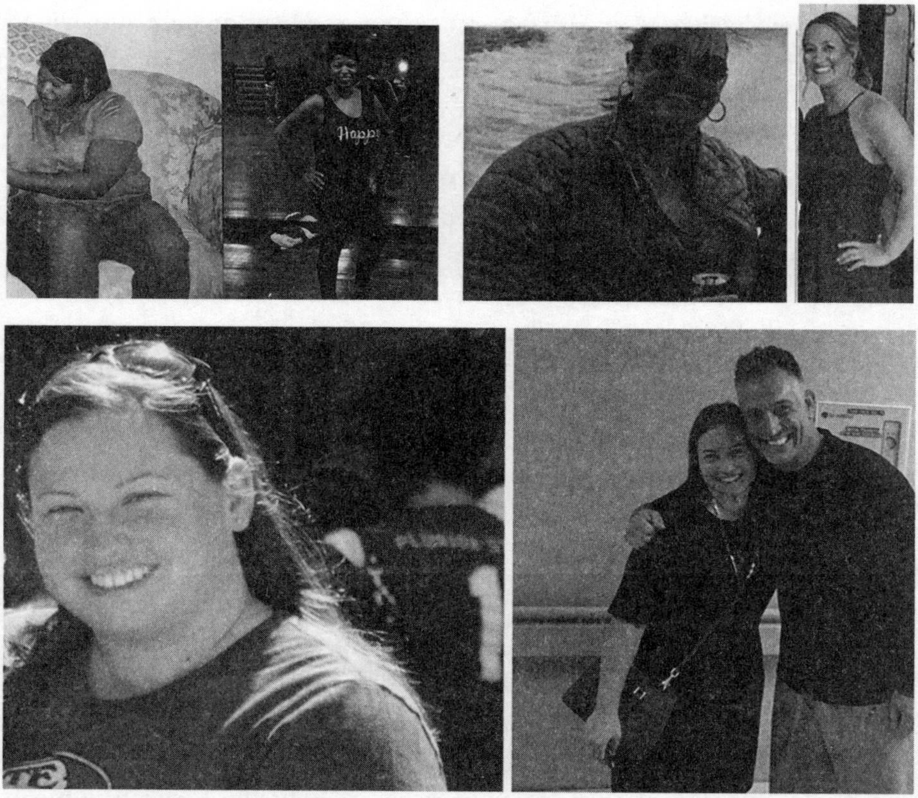

Three other patients who underwent freezing of the hunger nerve. All three reported significantly decreased hunger which allowed them to stick to their diet/exercise program of choice, which then fueled momentum and drove them through their Catching Points.

Medications are also available to ease the transition from overweight or obese to lean using diet and exercise. They are further evidence that a backlash is present when people try a new diet and/or exercise program, and is responsible for the current failure rate of at least 95 percent when folks try to lose weight on their own, and is exaggerated in the obese and overweight population such that they face a unique challenge when attempting weight loss. Available drug therapies for weight loss can be divided into the following classifications: (1) drugs for other conditions that cause weight gain (need to stop these), (2) drugs that mimic the actions of the satiety (fullness) hormones, (3) drugs that block the actions of the hunger hormones, (4) drugs that cause malabsorption, and (5) other.

Regarding the first of these, there are several common medications that obesity medicine physicians recognize and stop prescribing because of associated weight gain. Oftentimes these medications are prescribed by other physicians for legitimate reasons but can be replaced with a different drug that minimizes weight gain. Common examples include switching one blood pressure medication (often a class called beta blockers) for another, an adjustment that often results in immediate acceleration of weight loss. Other examples of medications patients often "walk in" on that contribute to weight gain and difficulty with weight loss are over-the-counter antihistamines or even herbal supplements.

Proven behavioral interventions actually underpin the entire catching point transformation program (and you thought I was making this stuff up). Specifically, there are five clear conclusions drawn from more than 50 years of observational and interventional research in this space. These conclusions serve as the framework for overcoming the body's resistance to dieting as follows.

First, something is better than nothing. Said another way, "progress, not perfection" is the preferable goal. Time and time again, the pursuit of perfection leads to failure. Inability to keep a predetermined schedule leads to the all-or-nothing decision to "quit your diet." Patients and the public should strive to accumulate as much change as possible in the long run. That is, successful weight loss will come for the person who is persistent about accumulating 15 progressive workouts or 15 healthy meals or 15 recoveries *in total, over any amount of time*, vs. hit-or-miss attempts at grandiose weight loss and transformation.

Second, flexibility is associated with success. Rigid structure leads to failure. People cannot follow static schedules for a host of reasons: the body rebels, life gets in the way, motivation wanes, and so on. The same principle applies to staying on track with regard to fitness, recovery, *and* diet.

Third, the hunger hormone system can be bypassed, and appetite can be changed. A complex system of hunger hormones exist that drives human beings to eat in order to survive. This system is responsible for the intense hunger pangs, fatigue, and motivation "zap" that follows the onset of calorie restriction and new exercise. This system can be modified through careful (intentional) activity and supplemented recovery to keep patients and the public on track.

Fourth, recovery is essential for actual body change to take place. Successful people in the fitness space attend to recovery. Obese individuals do not have the exercise capacity to significantly affect calorie balance. Exercise in this group can be utilized to induce adaption so that (1) individuals will improve, in a kinetic fashion, their ability to burn absolute calories, and (2) the body will initiate neural signals from the periphery to the brain, resulting in cortical (brain) reconstruction (change) that will ease the burden of exercise.

Fifth, an activity-mediated transformative approach to healthy living is possible. Lessons learned through the study of exercise biology point toward molecular modification through activity as a new frontier of healthy living. Essentially what this means is that a focus on improving exercise capacity and shifting protein metabolism to muscles will initiate global feedback mechanisms that accelerate long-term change. This is that change that creates the desire for clean eating and exercise.

APPENDIX 1—

Kinetic Change

THE TOOLS AND RECTANGLE boxes that we collect in between workouts are called kinetic energy or kinetic change. Strictly speaking, kinetic energy is the energy gained by a mass when it is accelerated from rest to a given velocity. I know that sounds a bit "blah, blah, blah," but bear with me. It means that at time 0:00, you—represented by a ball in the figures—are at rest. Making no progress toward anything. At time X, you are moving at some speed. Kinetic energy is the energy you gained going from rest to whatever speed you ended up at.

In the first figure, the ball has no speed and no kinetic energy. The workouts are how we normally measure our progress and correlate with speed in this example. At different workouts (1, 2, 3, etc.), the ball will measure different speeds, and in between each will have gained kinetic energy. It is this kinetic energy that we care about! We care about what happens in between workouts more than the workouts themselves because that is when the changes we want are occurring. You need to accumulate this kinetic energy and the changes in your body that go along with it in order to be successful.

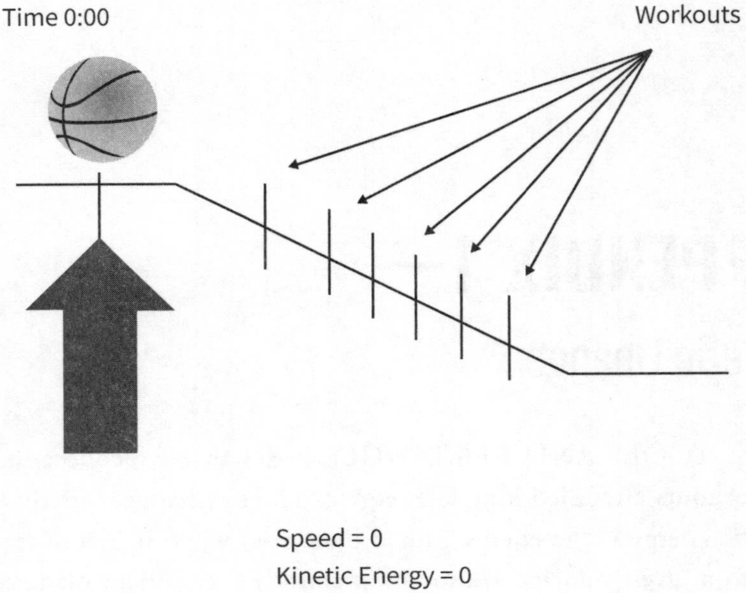
Time 0:00
Workouts
Speed = 0
Kinetic Energy = 0

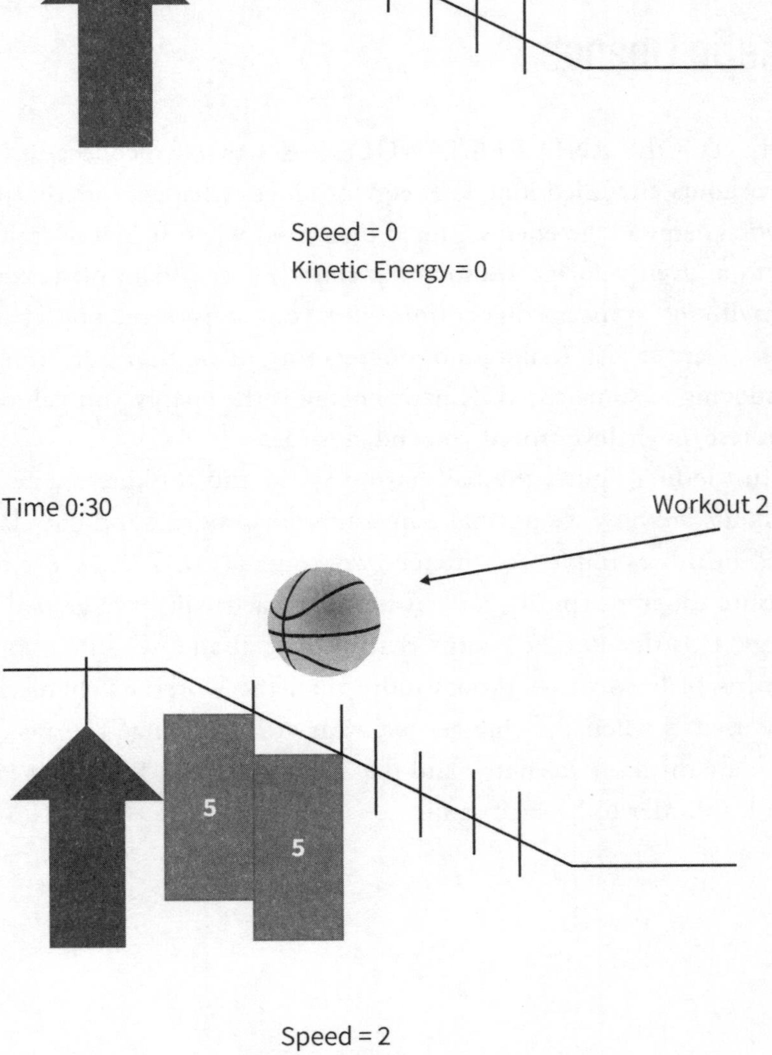
Time 0:30
Workout 2
5
5
Speed = 2
Kinetic Energy = 10

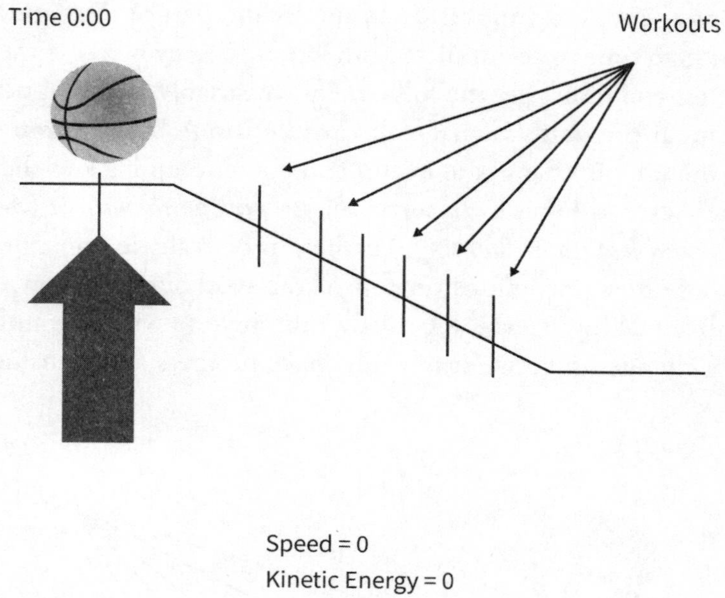
Time 0:00
Workouts
Speed = 0
Kinetic Energy = 0

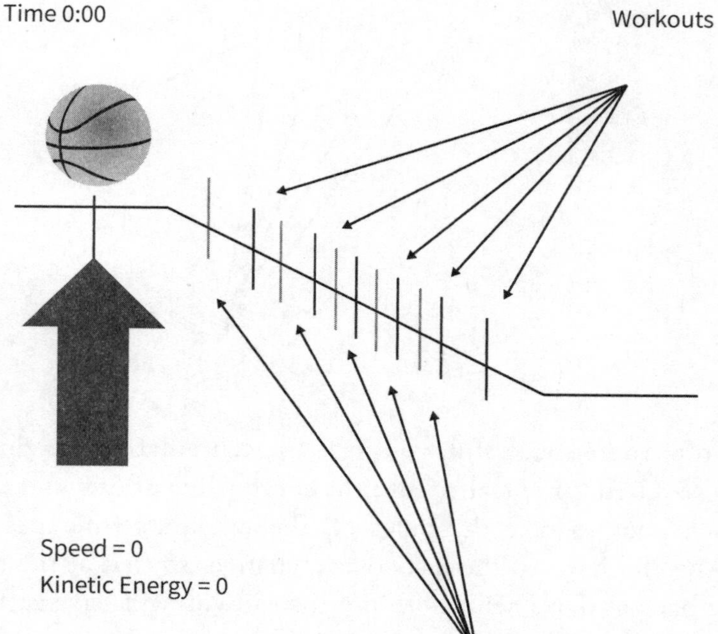
Time 0:00
Workouts
Speed = 0
Kinetic Energy = 0
Diet Restrictions

The problem is, as you can see in the second part of this figure, there wasn't enough time to accumulate both kinetic energy boxes so they overlapped, and you didn't get the full benefit. Invariably what happens next in traditional programs is that you can't continue because you haven't allowed the kinetic changes to occur, and you end up back at the beginning where everything is 0. *Importantly, you give up the kinetic energy you did create and leave with nothing.* Further, to be realistic, most programs superimpose diet restrictions on top of the workouts, as shown in the next figure, making it even less likely that anyone will accumulate the necessary changes in between to really make progress and transform.

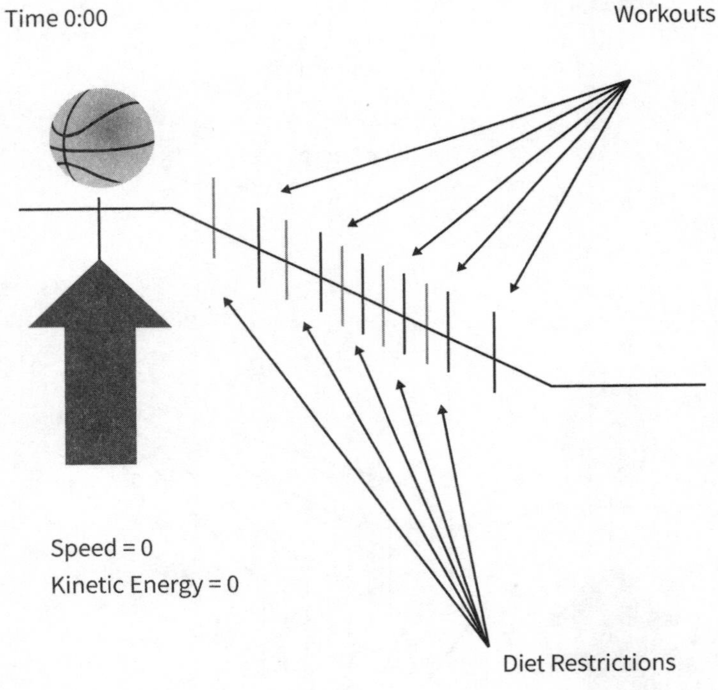

In order to be successful, you have to accumulate these changes—they are required for entrance into the success line of diet and exercise. This book aims to take the focus off the workouts (the speeds) and change the emphasis to the in-between changes so that at the end you won't be back at day 1 with nothing. Instead you will have accumulated the necessary kinetic energy (kinetic changes) to be successful long term with diet and exercise.

We move the workouts as necessary to maximize the kinetic energy gains. So if we started with the same idea, our program would deviate and finish differently, depending on the individual, so that our figures would look something like this:

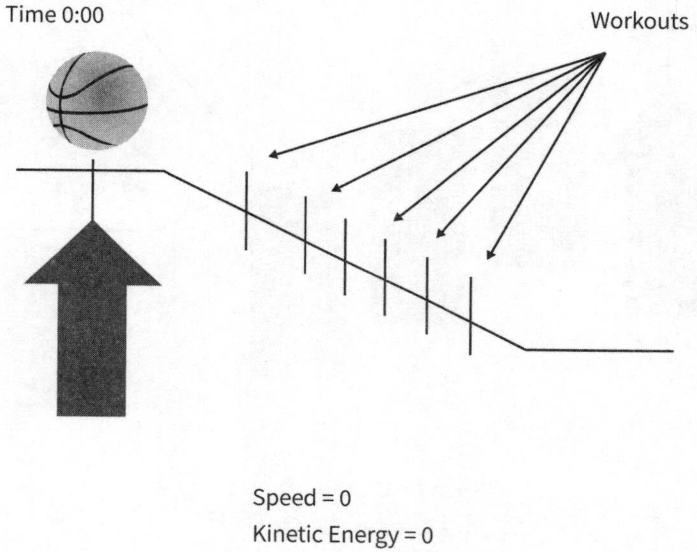

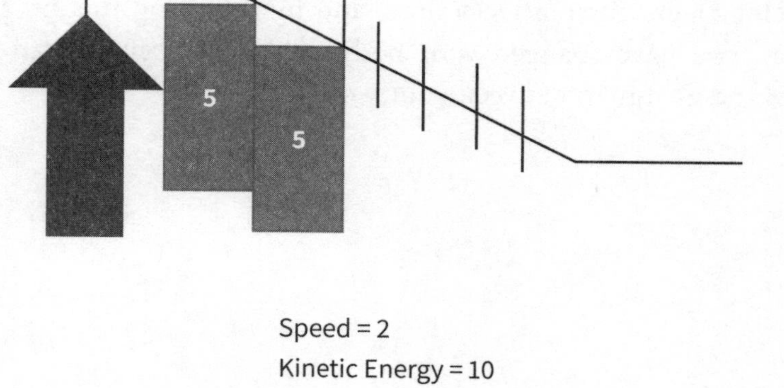

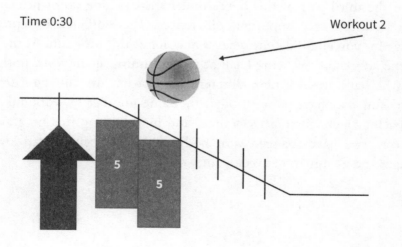

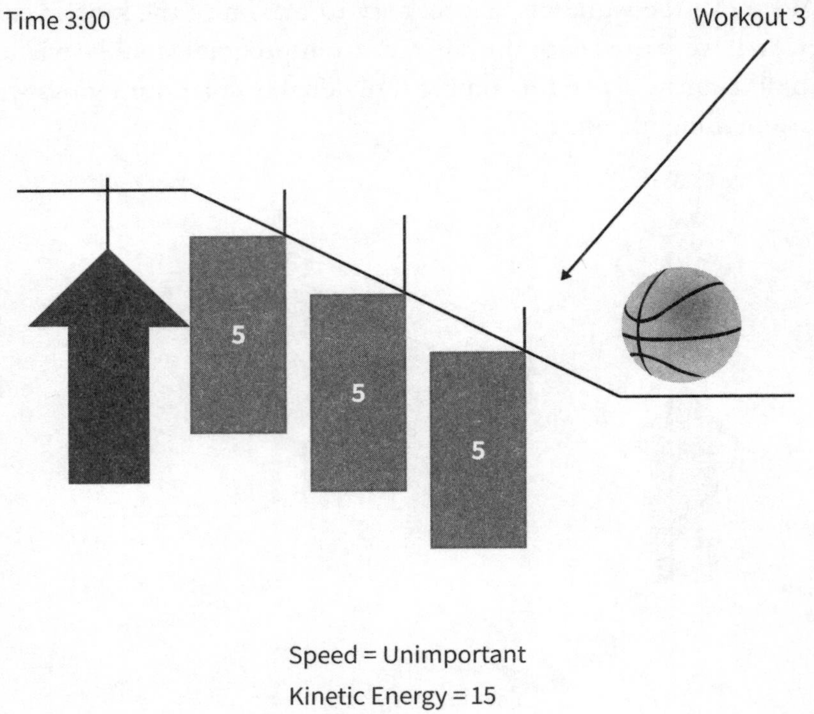

In the third part of this figure under the catching point principles, there are a few very important differences. These differences represent change for you and illustrate what is new about this program. At the end of time X, instead of being back at the beginning again, with nothing, you (the ball) are at a new, different place, what we call the catching point. You may have gone through the same number of workouts, but by spacing them differently in time, and by following this program in between, you have changed your body. You have accumulated kinetic changes and energy in between your workouts.

APPENDIX 2—

The Molecular Soldiers of Sleep

THE BENEFITS OF SLEEP, as it relates to exercise, weight loss, and fitness, can be divided broadly into two categories: recovery and the homeostasis of energy metabolism in humans. The first, recovery, is mediated through direct stimulation of protein transcription, through the production of antioxidant molecules, and through adjustment of immunological mediator profiles.[96, 97, 129, 204–207]

That is, exercise results in a disruption of our molecular structure, a disruption that the body will seek to correct—to replace with improved molecules and stronger structure. This new structure will have the capacity to endure a greater amount of exercise, thereby ultimately tipping the caloric balance. In order for this rebuilding to occur, though, growth hormone (GH) must mediate anabolic processes. It does so by inducing the liver to produce insulin growth-like factors (IGFs) that circulate and act on dormant cells to strengthen the body's framework and increase metabolism.[208–211] This is important for us so that we can increase metabolism, avoid injury, and improve our exercise capacity. *Growth hormone reaches its peaks during sleep.* When the body is sleep deprived, it switches to survival mode and foregoes optimization. As long as there is no apocalypse and we don't have to kill to survive and so forth, then we can optimize our physical status. In order to do so we must access this reorganization strategy, mediated by GH during sleep.

Similarly, the body will shut down our "fight or flight" response when adequately rested and turn on a parasympathetic response, which focuses inward on rebuilding. Otherwise, this response exists at a low level, which is counterproductive to our cause. In this situation, hormones and proteins, appropriately named "stress proteins" or "the stress response," circulate in relatively higher levels, resulting in increased storage of fat and toxicity to our muscles.[97, 108, 212, 213] Finally, in the absence of adequate sleep following exercise, the body exhibits a pro-inflammatory response, consisting of molecules called pro-inflammatory cytokines and characteristic immune cell presence, which causes direct damage to our body in addition to hindering our recovery.[102, 103, 107] Conversely, sleep is associated with decreased levels of all these mediators and uninterrupted re-organization of our underlying structure following exercise (figure A2a).

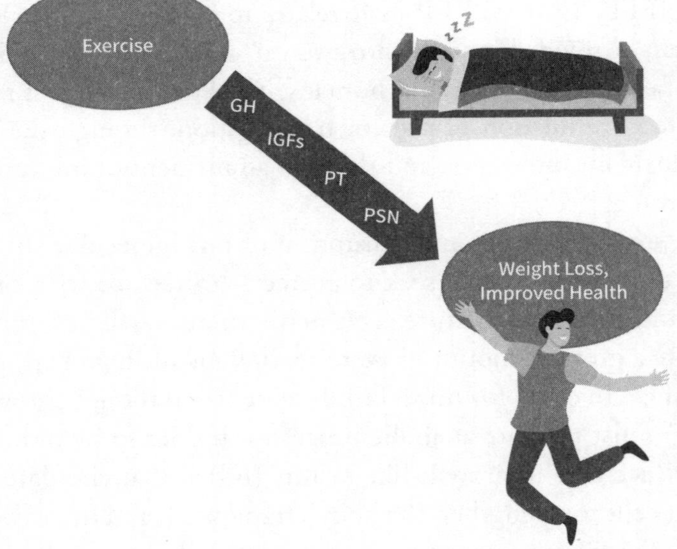

Figure A2a. In the presence of adequate rest, the body mediates change after exercise through growth hormone (GH), insulin-like growth factors (IGFs), muscle protein transcription (PT), and parasympathetic nervous system (PSN) activation.

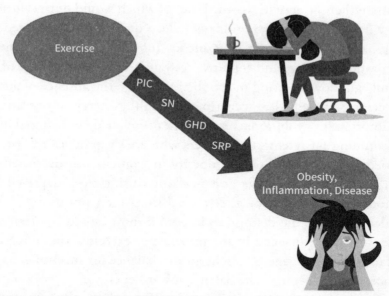

Figure A2b. In the absence of adequate rest, the body mediates change after exercise through proinflammatory cytokines (PIC), sympathetic nervous system activation (SN), growth hormone deficiency (GHD), and stress response proteins (SRP).

Secondly, sleep is intricately related to the energy cycle and homeostasis. As was the theme in many of the earlier chapters, the body's responses and adaptations are often rooted in evolution and survival. This one is no different. Humans originally needed to sleep, eat, and reproduce in order for the species to survive. As a result, a bidirectional hormonal system evolved such that satiety (being full) resulted in sleep. Sleep is required for humans to "protect brain cells from the damaging effect of reactive oxygen species, allow sufficient time for the repair or replacement of essential cellular components…and deal with other biochemical consequences of waking metabolic activity."[95, 112] Studies have shown that sleep deprivation results in decreased energy expenditure during the day. This is an attempt by the body to equalize the energy in/energy out balance disrupted by extensive waking hours. That is, the longer a person is awake, the more energy they are expending such that the body *then slows down metabolism and kicks out hunger hormones leading to increased intake* in an attempt to compensate.[112–114, 118, 214] Worse, the body would rather consume energy itself during sleep as part of the rebuilding process.[115]

What this means is that the body responds to less than optimal sleep duration by slowing metabolism, eating more, and foregoing rebuilding and strengthening activities—the latter of which would burn calories and energy itself! The same goes for poor sleep quality or interrupted sleep, which has also been shown to result in "increased hunger, uncontrolled and emotional eating, and cognitive restraint…as well as feelings of being less full" and lower resting metabolic rate.[214, 215] The absence of adequate sleep creates a paradoxical scenario of unhealthy energy conservation and consumption for evolutionary survival, a principle demonstrated in studies examining fat retention in dieters who are sleep deprived. The studies document worsened central obesity in women with decreased REM sleep, increased food intake and snacking during sleep-deprived states, and food-seeking behavior after partial sleep interruption.[116, 216] Figure A2c demonstrates the disruption in equilibrium caused by sleep disturbance, which is worsened in the presence of exercise. The human body seeks to equalize the energy in/energy out balance for survival at baseline. The absence of sleep tips the balance toward energy conservation, which translates to weight gain or, in our case, the blocking of weight loss.

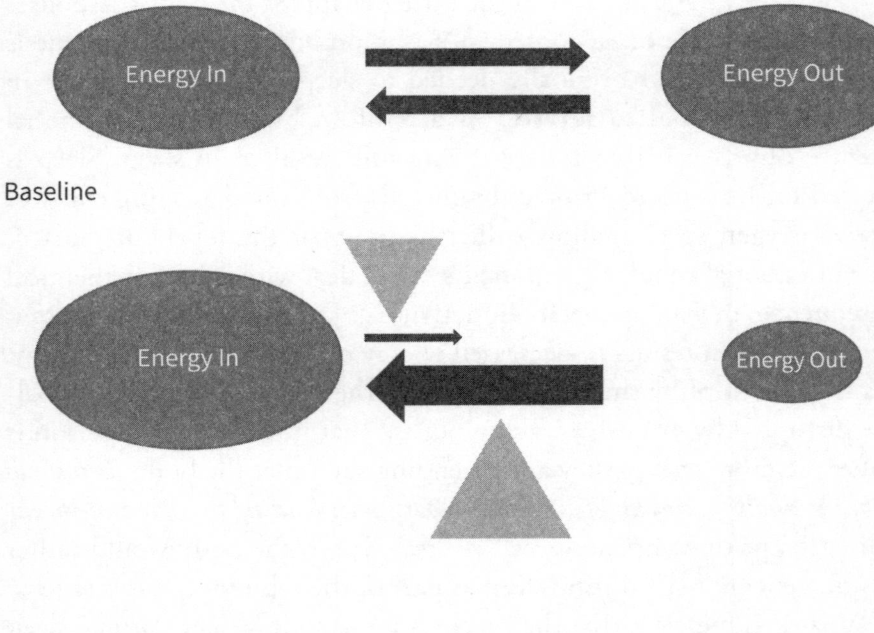

REFERENCES

1. Schutz, Y., and Abdul G Dulloo. "Resting metabolic rate, thermic effect of food, and obesity." In *Handbook of Obesity, edited by George A. Bray, 267.* Boca Raton, FL: CRC Press, 2014.

2. Davoodi, S.H., M. Ajami, S.A. Ayatollahi, K. Dowlatshahi, G. Javedan, H.R. Pazoki-Toroudi. "Calorie shifting diet versus calorie restriction diet: a comparative clinical trial study." *International Journal of Preventive Medicine* 5, no. 4 (2014):447–456.

3. Katz, David L., and Sean Lucan. *Nutrition in clinical practice.* Philadelphia, PA: LIppincott Williams and Wilkins, 2015.

4. Weiss, C.R., A.J. Gunn, C.Y. Kim, B.E. Paxton, D.L. Kraitchman, and A. Arepally. "Bariatric embolization of the gastric arteries for the treatment of obesity." *Journal of Vascular and Interventional Radiology* 26, no. 5 (2015):613–624.

5. Karra, E., A. Yousseif, R.L. Batterham. "Mechanisms facilitating weight loss and resolution of type 2 diabetes following bariatric surgery." *Trends in Endocrinology & Metabolism* 21, no. 6 (2010):337–344.

6. Chandarana, K., R.L. Batterham. "Shedding pounds after going under the knife: metabolic insights from cutting the gut." *Nature Medicine* 18 no. 5 (2012):668–669.

7. Howe, S.M., T.M. Hand, M.M. Manore. "Exercise-trained men and women: role of exercise and diet on appetite and energy intake." *Nutrients* 6, no. 11 (2014):4935–4960.

8. Gardiner, J.V., C.N. Jayasena, S.R. Bloom. "Gut hormones: a weight off your mind." *Journal of Neuroendocrinology* 20, no. 6 (2008):834–841.

9. Schubert, M.M., B. Desbrow, S. Sabapathy, M. Leveritt. "Acute exercise and hormones related appetite regulation: comparison of meta-analytical methods." *Sports Medicine* 44, no. 8 (2014):1167–1168.

10. Sainz, N., J. Barrenetxe, M.J. Moreno-Aliaga, J.A. Martinez. "Leptin resistance and diet-induced obesity: central and peripheral actions of leptin." *Metabolism* 64, no. 1 (2015):35–46.

11. Bluher, M., C.S. Mantzoros. "From leptin to other adipokines in health and disease: facts and expectations at the beginning of the 21st century. *Metabolism* 64, no. 1 (2015):131–145.

12. Borer, K.T. "Counterregulation of insulin by leptin as key component of autonomic regulation of body weight." *World Journal of Diabetes* 5, no. 5 (2014):606–629.

13. Murray, S., A. Tulloch, M.S. Gold, N.M. Avena. "Hormonal and neural mechanisms of food reward, eating behaviour and obesity." *Nature Reviews Endocrinology* 10, no. 9 (2014):540–552.

14. Bays, H. "Adiposopathy, "sick fat," Ockham's razor, and resolution of the obesity paradox." *Current Atherosclerosis Report* 16, no. 5 (2014):409.

15. Langin, D. "Adipose tissue metabolism, adipokines, and obesity." In *Handbook of Obesity, edited by George A. Bray, 225.* Boca Raton, FL: CRC Press, 2014, 2014.

16. Blouin, K., M. Nadeau, J.Mailloux, et al. "Pathways of adipose tissue androgen metabolism in women: depot differences and modulation by adipogenesis." *American Journal of Physiology Endocrinology and Metabolism* 296, no. 2 (2009):E244–255.

17. Cypess, A.M., S.Lehman, G.Williams, et al. "Identification and importance of brown adipose tissue in adult humans." *New England Journal of Medicine* 360, no. 15 (2009):1509–1517.

18. Backhed, F., H. Ding, T. Wang, et al. "The gut microbiota as an environmental factor that regulates fat storage." *Proceedings of the National Academy of Sciences of the USA* 101, no. 44 (2004):15718–15723.

19. Turnbaugh, P.J., R.E. Ley, M.A.Mahowald, V. Magrini, E.R.Mardis, J.I. Gordon. "An obesity-associated gut microbiome with increased capacity for energy harvest." *Nature* 444, no.7122 (2006):1027–1031.

20. Ley, R.E., P.J.Turnbaugh, S.Klein, J.I. Gordon. "Microbial ecology: human gut microbes associated with obesity." *Nature* 444, no. 7122 (2006):1022–1023.

21. Jayasinghe, TN., V. Chiavaroli, D.J.Holland, W.S.Cutfield, J.M. O'Sullivan. "The New Era of Treatment for Obesity and Metabolic Disorders: Evidence and Expectations for Gut Microbiome Transplantation." *Frontiers in Cellular and Infection Microbiology* 6 (2016):15.

22. Kolata, G. "The Science of Fat: After 'The Biggest Loser,' Their Bodies Fought to Regain Weight." *The New York Times*. May 2, 2016.

23. Rhodes, R.E., A Quinlan. "Predictors of physical activity change among adults using observational designs." *Sports Medicine* 45, no. 3 (2015):423–441.

24. Levi, J. "The State of Obesity: Better Policies for a Healthier America 2014." RWFJ, September 4, 2014.

25. Morton, J.P., A.C. Kayani, A. McArdle, B. Drust. "The exercise-induced stress response of skeletal muscle, with specific emphasis on humans." *Sports Medicine* 39, no. 8 (2009):643–662.

26. Svendsen, I.S., S.C. Killer, M. Gleeson. "Influence of Hydration Status on Changes in Plasma Cortisol, Leukocytes, and Antigen-Stimulated Cytokine Production by Whole Blood Culture following Prolonged Exercise." *International Scholarly Research Notices* 2014 (2014):1–10.

27. Coyle, E.F. "Physical activity as a metabolic stressor." *The American Journal of Clinical Nutrition* 72, suppl. 2 (2000):512S–520S.

28. Godin, R., A. Ascah, F.N. Daussin. "Intensity-dependent activation of intracellular signalling pathways in skeletal muscle: role of fibre type recruitment during exercise." *The Journal of Physiology* 588, no. 21 (2010):4073–4074.

29. Xing, J.Q., Y. Zhou, W. Fang, et al. "The effect of pre-competition training on biochemical indices and immune function of volleyball players." *International Journal of Clinical and Experimental Medicine* 6, no. 8 (2013):712–715.

30. Margaritelis, N.V., A. Kyparos, V. Paschalis, et al. "Reductive stress after exercise: The issue of redox individuality." *Redox biology* 2 (2014)520–528.

31. Astorino, T.A., M.M. Schubert. "Individual responses to completion of short-term and chronic interval training: a retrospective study." *PloS One* 9, no. 5 (2014):e97638.

32. Nascimento, Dda C., Rde C. Durigan, R.A. Tibana, J.L. Durigan, J.W. Navalta, J. Prestes. "The response of matrix metalloproteinase-9 and -2 to exercise." *Sports Medicine* 45, no. 2 (2015):269–278.

33. Mujika, I., S. Padilla, D. Pyne, T. Busso. "Physiological changes associated with the pre-event taper in athletes." *Sports Medicine* 34, no. 13 (2004):891–927.

34. Janikowska, G., A. Kochanska-Dziurowicz, A. Zebrowska, A. Bijak, M. Kimsa. "Adrenergic response to maximum exercise of trained road cyclists." *Journal of Human Kinetics* 40 (2014):103–111.

35. Pattyn, N., V.A. Cornelissen, S.R. Eshghi, L. Vanhees. "The effect of exercise on the cardiovascular risk factors constituting the metabolic syndrome: a meta-analysis of controlled trials." *Sports Medicine* 43, no. 2 (2013):121–133.

36. Menicucci, D., A. Piarulli, F. Mastorci, et al. "Interactions between immune, stress-related hormonal and cardiovascular systems following strenuous physical exercise." *Archives Italiennes de Biologie* 151 no. 3 (2013):126–136.

37. Phillips, S.M. "A brief review of critical processes in exercise-induced muscular hypertrophy." *Sports Medicine* 44 (2014):71–77.

38. Drygas, W., E. Rebowska, E. Stepien, J. Golanski, M. Kwasniewska. "Biochemical and hematological changes following the 120-km open-water marathon swim." *Journal of Sports Science & Medicine* 13, no. 3 (2014):632–637.

39. Buchheit, M., P.B. Laursen. "High-intensity interval training, solutions to the programming puzzle: Part I: cardiopulmonary emphasis." *Sports Medicine* 43, no. 5 (2013):313–338.

40. Neubauer, O., D. Konig, K.H. Wagner. "Recovery after an Ironman triathlon: sustained inflammatory responses and muscular stress." *European Journal of Applied Physiology* 104, no. 3 (2008):417–426.

41. Colvin, Geoffrey. *Talent is Overrated. What really separates world-class performers from everybody else.* New York, New York: Penguin Group, 2008.

42. Berthoud, H.R. "Homeostatic and non-homeostatic pathways involved in the control of food intake and energy balance." *Obesity* 14, suppl. 8 (2006):197S–200S.

43. Berthoud, H.R. "Neural control of appetite: cross-talk between homeostatic and non-homeostatic systems." *Appetite* 43, no. 3 (2004):315–317.

44. Weiss, C.R., A.J. Gunn, C.Y. Kim, B.E. Paxton, D.L. Kraitchman, A. Arepally. "Bariatric Embolization of the Gastric Arteries for the Treatment of Obesity." *Journal of Vascular and Interventional Radiology* 26, no. 5 (2015): 613–624.

45. Minett, G.M., R. Duffield. "Is recovery driven by central or peripheral factors? A role for the brain in recovery following intermittent-sprint exercise." *Frontiers in Physiology* 5. (2014):24.

46. Peinado, A.B., J.J. Rojo, F.J. Calderon, N. Maffulli. "Responses to increasing exercise upon reaching the anaerobic threshold, and their control by the central nervous system." *BMC Sports Science, Medicine and Rehabilitation* 6 (2014):17.

47. Kjaer, M., N.H Secher. "Neural influence on cardiovascular and endocrine responses to static exercise in humans." *Sports Medicine* 13, no. 5 (1992):303–319.

48. Beckman, L.M., T.R. Beckman, S.D. Sibley, et al. "Changes in gastrointestinal hormones and leptin after Roux-en-Y gastric bypass surgery." *JPEN Journal of Parenteral and Enteral Nutrition* 35, no. 2 (2011):169–180.

49. Disse, E., A.L. Bussier, N. Deblon, et al. "Systemic ghrelin and reward: effect of cholinergic blockade." *Physiology & Behavior* 102, no. 5 (2011):481–484.

50. Sobo, H. "Brains Response to High Fructose Corn Syrup May Explain Addiciton to Fast Foods." *Optimal Health Medical* (blog), March 2015.

51. Avena, N.M., S. Murray, M.S. Gold. "Comparing the effects of food restriction and overeating on brain reward systems." *Experimental Gerontology* 48, no. 10 (2013):1062–1067.

52. Lee, S., H.B. Kwak. "Effects of interventions on adiponectin and adiponectin receptors." *Journal of Exercise Rehabilitation* 10, no. 2 (2014):60–68.

53. Schalow, G., G.A. Zach. "Reorganization of the human central nervous system." *General Physiology and Biophysics* 19, no. S1 (2000):11–240.

54. Gowing, L., M.F. Farrell, R. Ali, J.M. White. "Alpha2-adrenergic agonists for the management of opioid withdrawal." *The Cochrane Database of Systematic Reviews* 3 (2014):CD002024.

55. Miller, D.K., A. Bowirrat, M. Manka, et al. "Acute intravenous synaptamine complex variant KB220 "normalizes" neurological dysregulation in patients during protracted abstinence from alcohol and opiates as observed using quantitative electroencephalographic and genetic analysis for reward polymorphisms: part 1, pilot study with 2 case reports." *Postgraduate Medicine* 122, no. 6 (2010):188–213.

56. Pirowska, A., T. Wloch, R. Nowobilski, M. Plaszewski, A. Hocini, D. Menager. "Phantom phenomena and body scheme after limb amputation: a literature review." *Neurologia i Neurochirurgia Polska* 48, no. 1 (2014):52–59.

57. Griffin, S.C., J.W. Tsao. "A mechanism-based classification of phantom limb pain." *Pain* 155, no. 11 (2014).

58. Moesker, A.A., H.W. Karl, A.M. Trescot. "Treatment of phantom limb pain by cryoneurolysis of the amputated nerve." *Pain Practice* 14, no. 1 (2014):52–56.

59. Weeks, S.R., V.C. Anderson-Barnes, J.W. Tsao. "Phantom limb pain: theories and therapies." *The Neurologist* 16, no. 5 (2010):277–286.

60. Subedi, B., G.T. Grossberg. "Phantom limb pain: mechanisms and treatment approaches." *Pain Research and Treatment* 2011 (2011):864605.

61. Foell, J., R. Bekrater-Bodmann, H. Flor, J. Cole. "Phantom limb pain after lower limb trauma: origins and treatments." *The International Journal of Lower Extremity Wounds* 10, no. 4 (2011):224–235.

62. Foell, J., R. Bekrater-Bodmann, M. Diers, H. Flor. "Mirror therapy for phantom limb pain: brain changes and the role of body representation." *European Journal of Pain* 18, no. 5 (2014):729–739.

63. MacIver, K., D.M. Lloyd, S. Kelly, N. Roberts, T. Nurmikko. "Phantom limb pain, cortical reorganization and the therapeutic effect of mental imagery." *Brain: a Journal of Neurology* 131, no. 8 (2008):2181–2191.

64. Reilly, K.T., A. Sirigu. "The motor cortex and its role in phantom limb phenomena." *The Neuroscientist: a Review Journal Bringing Neurobiology, Neurology and Psychiatry* 14, no. 2 (2008):195–202.

65. Bezzola, L., S. Merillat, C. Gaser, L. Jancke. "Training-induced neural plasticity in golf novices." *The Journal of Neuroscience: the Official Journal of the Society for Neuroscience* 31, no. 35 (2011):12444–12448.

66. Thomas, C., C.I. Baker. "Teaching an adult brain new tricks: a critical review of evidence for training-dependent structural plasticity in humans." *NeuroImage* 73 (2013):225–236.

67. Ludacris. "Number One Spot." Released 2004. Track 2 on *Red Lights District.* Columbia Records.

68. Areta, J.L., L.M. Burke, M.L. Ross, et al. "Timing and distribution of protein ingestion during prolonged recovery from resistance exercise alters myofibrillar protein synthesis." *The Journal of Physiology* 591, no. 9 (2013):2319–2331.

69. Witard, O.C., S.R. Jackman, L. Breen, K. Smith, A. Selby, K.D. Tipton. "Myofibrillar muscle protein synthesis rates subsequent to a meal in response to increasing doses of whey protein at rest and after resistance exercise." *The American Journal of Clinical Nutrition* 99, no. 1 (2014):86–95.

70. Engel, F., S. Hartel, M.O. Wagner, J. Strahler, K. Bos, B. Sperlich. "Hormonal, Metabolic and Cardiorespiratory Responses of Young and Adult Athletes to a Single Session of High Intensity Cycle Exercise." *Pediatric Exercise Science* (2014).

71. Talanian, J.L., S.D. Galloway, G.J. Heigenhauser, A. Bonen, L.L. Spriet. "Two weeks of high-intensity aerobic interval training increases the capacity for fat oxidation during exercise in women." *Journal of Applied Physiology* 102, no. 4 (2007):1439–1447.

72. Tee, J.C., A.N. Bosch, M.I. Lambert. "Metabolic consequences of exercise-induced muscle damage." *Sports Medicine* 37, no. 10 (2007):827–836.

73. Barnett, A. "Using recovery modalities between training sessions in elite athletes: does it help?" *Sports Medicine* 36, no. 9 (2006):781–796.

74. Ebbeling, C.B., P.M. Clarkson. "Exercise-induced muscle damage and adaptation." *Sports Medicine* 7, no. 4 (1989):207–234.

75. Koenig, R., J.R. Dickman, C. Kang, T. Zhang, Y.F. Chu, L.L. Ji. "Avenanthramide supplementation attenuates exercise-induced inflammation in postmenopausal women." *Nutrition Journal* 13 (2014):21.

76. Barnes, M.J. "Alcohol: impact on sports performance and recovery in male athletes." *Sports Medicine* 44, no. 7 (2014):909–919.

77. Osterberg, K.L., C.L. Melby. "Effect of acute resistance exercise on postexercise oxygen consumption and resting metabolic rate in young women." *International Journal of Sport Nutrition and Exercise Metabolism* 10, no. 1 (2000):71–81.

78. Melby, C., C. Scholl, G. Edwards, R. Bullough. "Effect of acute resistance exercise on postexercise energy expenditure and resting metabolic rate." *Journal of Applied Physiology* 75, no. 4 (1993):1847–1853.

79. Stiegler, P., A. Cunliffe. "The role of diet and exercise for the maintenance of fat-free mass and resting metabolic rate during weight loss." *Sports Medicine* 36, no. 3 (2006):239–262.

80. Bielinski, R., Y. Schutz, E. Jequier. "Energy metabolism during the postexercise recovery in man." *The American Journal of Clinical Nutrition* 42, no. 1 (1985):69–82.

81. Belz, A. "Dr. Oz: fast metabolism plan with two splurge days and healthy fat days." WellBuzz, November 2014. http://www.wellbuzz.com/dr-oz-diet/dr-oz-fast-metabolism-plan-two-splurge-days-healthy-fat-days/. Accessed December 8, 2014.

82. Shin, H.S., J.R. Ingram, A.T. McGill, S.D. Poppitt. "Lipids, CHOs, proteins: can all macronutrients put a 'brake' on eating?" *Physiology & Behavior* 120 (2013):114–123.

83. Stark, R., S.E. Ashley, Z.B. Andrews. "AMPK and the neuroendocrine regulation of appetite and energy expenditure." *Molecular and Cellular Endocrinology* 366, no. 2 (2013):215–223.

84. Chanda, M.L., D.J. Levitin. "The neurochemistry of music." *Trends in Cognitive Sciences* 17, no. 4 (2013):179–193.

85. Cervellin, G., G. Lippi. "From music-beat to heart-beat: a journey in the complex interactions between music, brain and heart." *European Journal of Internal Medicine* 22, no. 4 (2011):371–374.

86. McGrane, N., R. Galvin, T. Cusack, E. Stokes. "Addition of motivational interventions to exercise and traditional Physiotherapy: a review and meta-analysis." *Physiotherapy* (2014).

87. Knicker, A.J., I. Renshaw, A.R. Oldham, S.P. Cairns. "Interactive processes link the multiple symptoms of fatigue in sport competition." *Sports Medicine* 41, no. 4 (2011):307–328.

88. Morelli, V., C. Davis. "The potential role of sports psychology in the obesity epidemic." *Primary Care* 40, no. 2 (2013):507–523.

89. Lehmann, M., H.H. Dickhuth, G. Gendrisch, et al. "Training-overtraining. A prospective, experimental study with experienced middle- and long-distance runners." *International Journal of Sports Medicine* 12, no. 5 (1991):444–452.

90. Hooper, S.L., L.T. Mackinnon, A. Howard, R.D. Gordon, A.W. Bachmann. "Markers for monitoring overtraining and recovery." *Medicine and Science in Sports and Exercise* 27, no. 1 (1995):106–112.

91. Hooper, S.L., L.T. Mackinnon. "Monitoring overtraining in athletes. Recommendations." *Sports Medicine* 20, no. 5 (1995):321–327.

92. Lewis, N.A., G. Howatson, K. Morton, J. Hill, C.R. Pedlar. "Alterations in redox homeostasis in the elite endurance athlete." *Sports Medicine* 45, no. 3 (2015):379–409.

93. Saw, A.E., L.C. Main, P.B. Gastin. "The role of a self-report measure in athlete preparation." *Journal of Strength and Conditioning Research: National Strength & Conditioning Association* (2014).

94. Nedelec, M., A. McCall, C. Carling, F. Legall, S. Berthoin, G. Dupont. "Recovery in soccer: part I - post-match fatigue and time course of recovery." *Sports Medicine* 42, no. 12 (2012):997–1015.

95. Siegel, J.M. "Clues to the functions of mammalian sleep." *Nature* 437, no. 7063 (2005):1264–1271.

96. Dattilo, M., H.K. Antunes, A. Medeiros, et al. "Sleep and muscle recovery: endocrinological and molecular basis for a new and promising hypothesis." *Medical Hypotheses* 77, no. 2 (2011):220–222.

97. Demarzo, M.M., P.K. Stein. "Mental Stress and Exercise Training Response: Stress-sleep Connection may be Involved." *Frontiers in Physiology* 3. (2012):178.

98. Kalsbeek, A., S. la Fleur, E. Fliers. "Circadian control of glucose metabolism." *Molecular Metabolism* 3, no. 4 (2014):372–383.

99. Spiegel, K., R. Leproult, E. Van Cauter. "Impact of sleep debt on metabolic and endocrine function." *Lancet* 354, no. 9188 (1999):1435–1439.

100. Irwin, M.R. "Why Sleep Is Important for Health: A Psychoneuroimmunology Perspective." *Annual Review of Psychology* 66 (2014).

101. Irwin, M.R., R.E. Olmstead, P.A. Ganz, R. Haque. "Sleep disturbance, inflammation and depression risk in cancer survivors." *Brain, Behavior, and Immunity* 30, suppl. (2013):S58–67.

102. Thomas, K.S., S. Motivala, R. Olmstead, M.R. Irwin. "Sleep depth and fatigue: role of cellular inflammatory activation." *Brain, Behavior, and Immunity* 25, no. 1 (2011):53–58.

103. Vgontzas, A.N., E. Zoumakis, E.O. Bixler, et al. "Adverse effects of modest sleep restriction on sleepiness, performance, and inflammatory cytokines." *The Journal of Clinical Endocrinology and Metabolism* 89, no. 5 (2004):2119–2126.

104. Bahijri, S., A. Borai, G. Ajabnoor, et al. "Relative metabolic stability, but disrupted circadian cortisol secretion during the fasting month of Ramadan." *PloS One* 8, no. 4 (2013):e60917.

105. Clevenger, L., A. Schrepf, D. Christensen, et al. "Sleep disturbance, cytokines, and fatigue in women with ovarian cancer." *Brain, Behavior, and Immunity* 26, no. 7 (2012):1037–1044.

106. Perry, G.S., S.P. Patil, L.R. Presley-Cantrell. "Raising awareness of sleep as a healthy behavior." *Preventing Chronic Disease* 10. (2013):E133.

107. Liu, L., P.J. Mills, M. Rissling, et al. "Fatigue and sleep quality are associated with changes in inflammatory markers in breast cancer patients undergoing chemotherapy." *Brain, Behavior, and Immunity* 26, no. 5 (2012):706–713.

108. Meier-Ewert, H.K., P.M. Ridker, N. Rifai, et al. "Effect of sleep loss on C-reactive protein, an inflammatory marker of cardiovascular risk." *Journal of the American College of Cardiology* 43, no. 4 (2004):678–683.

109. Anafi, R.C., R. Pellegrino, K.R. Shockley, M. Romer, S. Tufik, A.I. Pack. "Sleep is not just for the brain: transcriptional responses to sleep in peripheral tissues." *BMC Genomics* 14. (2013):362.

110. Strazzullo, P., L. D'Elia, G. Cairella, F. Garbagnati, F.P. Cappuccio, L. Scalfi. "Excess body weight and incidence of stroke: meta-analysis of prospective studies with 2 million participants." *Stroke: a Journal of Cerebral Circulation* 41, no. 5 (2010):e418–426.

111. Fullagar, H.H., S. Skorski, R. Duffield, D. Hammes, A.J. Coutts, T. Meyer. "Sleep and athletic performance: the effects of sleep loss on exercise performance, and physiological and cognitive responses to exercise." *Sports Medicine* 45, no. 2 (2015):161–186.

112. Vanitallie, T.B. "Sleep and energy balance: Interactive homeostatic systems." *Metabolism: Clinical and Experimental* 55, suppl. 2 (2006):S30–35.

113. Nicolaidis, S. "Metabolic mechanism of wakefulness (and hunger) and sleep (and satiety): Role of adenosine triphosphate and hypocretin and other peptides." *Metabolism: Clinical and Experimental* 55, suppl. 2 (2006):S24–29.

114. Gallagher, T., Y.J. You. "Falling asleep after a big meal: Neuronal regulation of satiety." *Worm* 3. (2014):e27938.

115. Wong-Riley, M. "What is the meaning of the ATP surge during sleep?" *Sleep* 34, no. 7 (2011):833–834.

116. Nedeltcheva, A.V., J.M. Kilkus, J. Imperial, D.A. Schoeller, P.D. Penev. "Insufficient sleep undermines dietary efforts to reduce adiposity." *Annals of Internal Medicine* 153, no. 7 (2010):435–441.

117. Taheri, S., E. Mignot. "Sleep well and stay slim: dream or reality?" *Annals of Internal Medicine* 153, no. 7 (2010):475–476.

118. Calvin, A.D., R.E. Carter, T. Adachi, et al. "Effects of experimental sleep restriction on caloric intake and activity energy expenditure." *Chest* 144, no. 1 (2013):79–86.

119. St-Onge, M.P., A. McReynolds, Z.B. Trivedi, A.L. Roberts, M. Sy, J. Hirsch. "Sleep restriction leads to increased activation of brain regions sensitive to food stimuli." *The American Journal of Clinical Nutrition* 95, no. 4 (2012):818–824.

120. Chaput, J.P., L. Klingenberg, A.M. Sjodin. "Sleep restriction and appetite control: waking to a problem?" *The American Journal of Clinical Nutrition* 91, no. 3 (2010):822–823; author reply 823–824.

121. Pejovic, S., A.N. Vgontzas, M. Basta, et al. "Leptin and hunger levels in young healthy adults after one night of sleep loss." *Journal of Sleep Research* 19, no. 4 (2010):552–558.

122. Chapman, C.D., C. Benedict, S.J. Brooks, H.B. Schioth. "Lifestyle determinants of the drive to eat: a meta-analysis." *The American Journal of Clinical Nutrition* 96, no. 3 (2012):492–497.

123. Brondel, L., M.A. Romer, P.M. Nougues, P. Touyarou, D. Davenne. "Acute partial sleep deprivation increases food intake in healthy men." *The American Journal of Clinical Nutrition* 91, no. 6 (2010):1550–1559.

124. Spaeth, A.M., D.F. Dinges, N. Goel. "Effects of Experimental Sleep Restriction on Weight Gain, Caloric Intake, and Meal Timing in Healthy Adults." *Sleep* 36, no. 7 (2013):981–990.

125. St-Onge, M.P., S. Wolfe, M. Sy, A. Shechter, J. Hirsch. "Sleep restriction increases the neuronal response to unhealthy food in normal-weight individuals." *International Journal of Obesity* 38, no. 3 (2014):411–416.

126. Cappuccio, F.P., L. D'Elia, P. Strazzullo, M.A. Miller. "Sleep duration and all-cause mortality: a systematic review and meta-analysis of prospective studies." *Sleep* 33, no. 5 (2010):585–592.

127. Cappuccio, F.P., D. Cooper, L. D'Elia, P. Strazzullo, M.A. Miller. "Sleep duration predicts cardiovascular outcomes: a systematic review and meta-analysis of prospective studies." *European Heart Journal* 32, no. 12 (2011):1484–1492.

128. Slattery, K., D. Bentley, A.J. Coutts. "The role of oxidative, inflammatory and neuroendocrinological systems during exercise stress in athletes: implications of antioxidant supplementation on physiological adaptation during intensified physical training." *Sports Medicine* 45, no. 4 (2015):453–471.

129. Halson, S.L. "Sleep in elite athletes and nutritional interventions to enhance sleep." *Sports Medicine* 44, suppl. 1 (2014):S13–23.

130. Res, P.T., B. Groen, B. Pennings, et al. "Protein ingestion before sleep improves postexercise overnight recovery." *Medicine and Science in Sports and Exercise* 44, no. 8 (2012):1560–1569.

131. Noble, E.G., K.J. Milne, C.W. Melling. "Heat shock proteins and exercise: a primer." *Applied Physiology, Nutrition, and Metabolism = Physiologie Appliquee, Nutrition et Metabolisme* 33, no. 5 (2008):1050–1065.

132. Liu, J., S.H. Jia, M. Kirberger, N. Chen. "Lunasin as a promising health-beneficial peptide." *European Review for Medical and Pharmacological Sciences* 18, no. 14 (2014):2070–2075.

133. Ortiz-Martinez, M., R. Winkler, S. Garcia-Lara. "Preventive and therapeutic potential of peptides from cereals against cancer." *Journal of Proteomics* 111 (2014).

134. Jeong, H.J., J.R. Lee, J.B. Jeong, J.H. Park, Y.K. Cheong, B.O. de Lumen. "The cancer preventive seed peptide lunasin from rye is bioavailable and bioactive." *Nutrition and Cancer* 61, no. 5 (2009):680–686.

135. de Lumen, B.O. "Lunasin: a cancer-preventive soy peptide." *Nutrition Reviews* 63, no. 1 (2005):16–21.

136. Hsieh, C.C., B. Hernandez-Ledesma, H.J. Jeong, J.H. Park, B.O. de Lumen. "Complementary roles in cancer prevention: protease inhibitor makes the cancer preventive peptide lunasin bioavailable." *PloS One* 5, no. 1 (2010):e8890.

137. Chen, Y.Y., M.H. Lai, H.Y. Hung, J.F. Liu. "Sweet potato [Ipomoea batatas (L.) Lam. "Tainong 57"] starch improves insulin sensitivity in high-fructose diet-fed rats by ameliorating adipocytokine levels, pro-inflammatory status, and insulin signaling." *Journal of Nutritional Science and Vitaminology* 59, no. 4 (2013):272–280.

138. Chang, W.H., S.P. Hu, Y.F. Huang, T.S. Yeh, J.F. Liu. "Effect of purple sweet potato leaves consumption on exercise-induced oxidative stress and IL-6 and HSP72 levels." *Journal of Applied Physiology* 109, no. 6 (2010):1710–1715.

139. Chao, P.Y., Y.P. Huang, W.B. Hsieh. "Inhibitive effect of purple sweet potato leaf extract and its components on cell adhesion and inflammatory response in human aortic endothelial cells." *Cell Adhesion & Migration* 7, no. 2 (2013):237–245.

140. Slattery, K., D. Bentley, A.J. Coutts. "The Role of Oxidative, Inflammatory and Neuroendocrinological Systems During Exercise Stress in Athletes: Implications of Antioxidant Supplementation on Physiological Adaptation During Intensified Physical Training." *Sports Medicine* 45 (2014).

141. Kono, H., K.L. Rock. "How dying cells alert the immune system to danger." *Nature Reviews Immunology* 8, no. 4 (2008):279–289.

142. Bozaykut, P., N.K. Ozer, B. Karademir. "Regulation of protein turnover by heat shock proteins." *Free Radical Biology & Medicine* (2014).

143. Lanneau, D., G. Wettstein, P. Bonniaud, C. Garrido. "Heat shock proteins: cell protection through protein triage." *The Scientific World Journal* 10 (2010):1543–1552.

144. Reid, J. "How to Make Buildings and Structures Earthquake Proof." Reid Steel, 2014. Accessed December 1, 2014.

145. Diplock, A.T., J.L. Charleux, G. Crozier-Willi, et al. "Functional food science and defence against reactive oxidative species." *The British Journal of Nutrition* 80, suppl. 1 (1998):S77–112.

146. Fernandes, A.P., V. Gandin. "Selenium compounds as therapeutic agents in cancer." *Biochimica et Biophysica Acta* 1850, no. 8 (2014).

147. Berkoff, F., S.J. *Foods that Harm Foods that Heal.* New York, New York: Trusted Media Brands, 2013.

148. Wu, H., A. Pan, Z. Yu, et al. "Lifestyle counseling and supplementation with flaxseed or walnuts influence the management of metabolic syndrome." *The Journal of Nutrition* 140, no. 11 (2010):1937–1942.

149. Bao, Y., J. Han, F.B. Hu, et al. "Association of nut consumption with total and cause-specific mortality." *The New England Journal of Medicine* 369, no. 21 (2013):2001–2011.

150. Falasca, M., I. Casari, T. Maffucci. "Cancer chemoprevention with nuts." *Journal of the National Cancer Institute* 106, no. 9 (2014).

151. Chen, S., H. Zhang, H. Pu, et al. "n-3 PUFA supplementation benefits microglial responses to myelin pathology." *Scientific Reports* 4 (2014):7458.

152. Abedi, E., M.A. Sahari. "Long-chain polyunsaturated fatty acid sources and evaluation of their nutritional and functional properties." *Food Science & Nutrition* 2, no. 5 (2014):443–463.

153. De Caterina, R., A. Zampolli, S. Del Turco, R. Madonna, M. Massaro. "Nutritional mechanisms that influence cardiovascular disease." *The American Journal of Clinical Nutrition* 83, suppl. 2 (2006):421S–426S.

154. Trio, P.Z., S. You, X. He, J. He, K. Sakao, D.X. Hou. "Chemopreventive functions and molecular mechanisms of garlic organosulfur compounds." *Food & Function* 5, no. 5 (2014):833–844.

155. Mason, S., G.D. Wadley. "Skeletal muscle reactive oxygen species: a target of good cop/bad cop for exercise and disease." *Redox Report: Communications in Free Radical Research* 19, no. 3 (2014):97–106.

156. Hausswirth, C., Y. Le Meur. "Physiological and nutritional aspects of post-exercise recovery: specific recommendations for female athletes." *Sports Medicine* 41, no. 10 (2011):861–882.

157. Beelen, M., L.M. Burke, M.J. Gibala, L.J. van Loon. "Nutritional strategies to promote postexercise recovery." *International Journal of Sport Nutrition and Exercise Metabolism* 20, no. 6 (2010;):515–532.

158. Finger, D, F.R. Goltz, D. Umpierre, E. Meyer, L.H. Rosa, C.D. Schneider. "Effects of protein supplementation in older adults undergoing resistance training: a systematic review and meta-analysis." *Sports Medicine* 45, no. 2 (2015):245–255.

159. Burd, N.A., J.E. Tang, D.R. Moore, S.M. Phillips. "Exercise training and protein metabolism: influences of contraction, protein intake, and sex-based differences." *Journal of Applied Physiology* 106, no. 5 (2009):1692–1701.

160. Koopman, R., A.J. Wagenmakers, R.J. Manders, et al. "Combined ingestion of protein and free leucine with carbohydrate increases postexercise muscle protein synthesis in vivo in male subjects." *American Journal of Physiology Endocrinology and Metabolism* 288, no. 4 (2005):E645–653.

161. Keller, U., G. Szinnai, S. Bilz, K. Berneis. "Effects of changes in hydration on protein, glucose and lipid metabolism in man: impact on health." *European Journal of Clinical Nutrition* 57, suppl. 2 (2003):S69–74.

162. Shahidi, F., J. McDonald, A. Chandrasekara, Y. Zhong. "Phytochemicals of foods, beverages and fruit vinegars: chemistry and health effects." *Asia Pacific Journal of Clinical Nutrition 17, no.* 1 (2008):380–382.

163. Liljeberg, H., I. Bjorck. "Delayed gastric emptying rate may explain improved glycaemia in healthy subjects to a starchy meal with added vinegar." *European Journal of Clinical Nutrition* 52, no. 5 (1998):368–371.

164. Ostman, E., Y. Granfeldt, L. Persson, I. Bjorck. "Vinegar supplementation lowers glucose and insulin responses and increases satiety after a bread meal in healthy subjects." *European Journal of Clinical Nutrition* 59, no. 9 (2005):983–988.

165. O'Keefe, J.H., N.M. Gheewala, J.O. O'Keefe. "Dietary strategies for improving post-prandial glucose, lipids, inflammation, and cardiovascular health." *Journal of the American College of Cardiology* 51, no. 3 (2008):249–255.

166. Yu, B.L., S.P. Zhao, J.R. Hu. "Cholesterol imbalance in adipocytes: a possible mechanism of adipocytes dysfunction in obesity." *Obesity Reviews: an Official Journal of the International Association for the Study of Obesity* 11, no. 8 (2010):560–567.

167. Wang, Z.Q., X.H. Zhang, J.C. Russell, M. Hulver, W.T. Cefalu. "Chromium picolinate enhances skeletal muscle cellular insulin signaling in vivo in obese, insulin-resistant JCR:LA-cp rats." *The Journal of Nutrition* 136, no. 2 (2006):415–420.

168. Lewicki, S., R. Zdanowski, M. Krzyzowska, et al. "The role of Chromium III in the organism and its possible use in diabetes and obesity treatment." *Annals of Agricultural and Environmental Medicine: AAEM* 21, no. 2 (2014):331–335.

169. Debarnot, U., M. Sperduti, F. Di Rienzo, A. Guillot. "Experts bodies, experts minds: How physical and mental training shape the brain." *Frontiers in Human Neuroscience* 8 (2014):280.

170. Knaepen, K., M. Goekint, E.M. Heyman, R. Meeusen. "Neuroplasticity - exercise-induced response of peripheral brain-derived neurotrophic factor: a systematic review of experimental studies in human subjects." *Sports Medicine* 40, no. 9 (2010):765–801.

171. Skriver, K., M. Roig, J. Lundbye-Jensen, et al. "Acute exercise improves motor memory: Exploring potential biomarkers." *Neurobiology of Learning and Memory* 116 (2014):46–58.

172. Taylor, A.G., L.E. Goehler, D.I. Galper, K.E. Innes, C. Bourguignon. "Top-down and bottom-up mechanisms in mind-body medicine: development of an integrative framework for psychophysiological research." *Explore* 6, no. 1 (2010):29–41.

173. Philips, M.F., G. Mattiasson, T. Wieloch, et al. "Neuroprotective and behavioral efficacy of nerve growth factor-transfected hippocampal progenitor cell transplants after experimental traumatic brain injury." *Journal of Neurosurgery* 94, no. 5 (2001):765–774.

174. Pal, R., S.N. Singh, K. Halder, O.S. Tomer, A.B. Mishra, M. Saha. "Effects of Yogic Practice on Metabolism and Antioxidant - Redox Status of Physically Active Males." *Journal of Physical Activity & Health* (2014).

175. Mahagita, C. "Roles of meditation on alleviation of oxidative stress and improvement of antioxidant system." *Journal of the Medical Association of Thailand = Chotmaihet thangphaet* 93, suppl. 6 (2010):S242–254.

176. Sharma, H., S. Sen, A. Singh, N.K. Bhardwaj, V. Kochupillai, N. Singh. "Sudarshan Kriya practitioners exhibit better antioxidant status and lower blood lactate levels." *Biological Psychology* 63, no. 3 (2003):281–291.

177. Sinha, S., S.N. Singh, Y.P. Monga, U.S. Ray. "Improvement of glutathione and total antioxidant status with yoga." *Journal of Alternative and Complementary Medicine* 13, no. 10 (2007):1085–1090.

178. Bauer, B. "Mind-Body Medicine at the Mayo Clinic." *Explore* 4, no. 5 (2008):295–299.

179. Srinivasan, T. "Bridging the mind-body divide." *International Journal of Yoga* 6, no. 2 (2013):85–86.

180. Nakata, H., K. Sakamoto, R. Kakigi. "Meditation reduces pain-related neural activity in the anterior cingulate cortex, insula, secondary somatosensory cortex, and thalamus." *Frontiers in Psychology* 5 (2014):1489.

181. Saatcioglu, F. "Regulation of gene expression by yoga, meditation and related practices: a review of recent studies." *Asian Journal of Psychiatry* 6, no. 1 (2013):74–77.

182. Pullen, P.R., S.H. Nagamia, P.K. Mehta, et al. "Effects of yoga on inflammation and exercise capacity in patients with chronic heart failure." *Journal of Cardiac Failure* 14, no. 5 (2008):407–413.

183. Anderson, J.G., A.G. Taylor. "The metabolic syndrome and mind-body therapies: a systematic review." *Journal of Nutrition and Metabolism* 2011 (2011):276419.

184. Felstead, C. *Yoga for runners.* Champaign, IL: Human Kinetics, 2014.

185. Hanh, T. *The Miracle of Mindfulness.* Boston, MA: Beacon Press, 1975.

186. Younge, J.O., R.A. Gotink, C.P. Baena, J.W. Roos-Hesselink, M.M. Hunink. "Mind-body practices for patients with cardiac disease: a systematic review and meta-analysis." *European Journal of Preventive Cardiology* 22, no. 11 (2014).

187. Carlson, C.R., R.H. Hoyle. "Efficacy of abbreviated progressive muscle relaxation training: a quantitative review of behavioral medicine research." *Journal of Consulting and Clinical Psychology* 61, no.6 (1993):1059–1067.

188. Hakkinen, K., M. Alen, M. Kallinen, R.U. Newton, W.J. Kraemer. "Neuromuscular adaptation during prolonged strength training, detraining and re-strength-training in middle-aged and elderly people." *European Journal of Applied Physiology* 83, no. 1 (2000):51–62.

189. Rapaport, M.H., P. Schettler, C. Bresee. "A preliminary study of the effects of repeated massage on hypothalamic-pituitary-adrenal and immune function in healthy individuals: a study of mechanisms of action and dosage." *Journal of Alternative and Complementary Medicine* 18, no.8 (2012):789–797.

190. Wiest, K.L., V.J. Asphaug, K.E. Carr, E.A. Gowen, T.T. Hartnett. "Massage Impact on Pain in Opioid-dependent Patients in Substance Use Treatment." *International Journal of Therapeutic Massage & Bodywork* 8, no. 1 (2015):12–24.

191. Lee, S.H., J.Y. Kim, S. Yeo, S.H. Kim, S. Lim. "Meta-Analysis of Massage Therapy on Cancer Pain." *Integrative Cancer Therapies* 14, no. 4 (2015).

192. Menetrier, A., L. Mourot, B. Degano, et al. "Effects of three post-exercice recovery treatments on femoral artery blood flow kinetics." *The Journal of Sports Medicine and Physical Fitness* (2014).

193. Born, D.P., B. Sperlich, H.C. Holmberg. "Bringing light into the dark: effects of compression clothing on performance and recovery." *International Journal of Sports Physiology and Performance* 8, no. 1 (2013):4–18.

194. Versey, N.G., S.L. Halson, B.T. Dawson. "Water immersion recovery for athletes: effect on exercise performance and practical recommendations." *Sports Medicine* 43, no. 11 (2013):1101–1130.

195. Bleakley, C.M., G.W. Davison. "What is the biochemical and physiological rationale for using cold-water immersion in sports recovery? A systematic review." *British Journal of Sports Medicine* 44, no. 3 (2010):179–187.

196. Vaile J, S. Halson, N. Gill, B. Dawson. "Effect of hydrotherapy on the signs and symptoms of delayed onset muscle soreness." *European Journal of Applied Physiology* 102, no. 4 (2008):447–455.

197. DL, K. "Lifestyle is the medicine, culture is the spoon: the covariance of proposition and preposition." *American Journal of Lifestyle Medicine* 8, no. 5 (2014):301–305.

198. Pagano, M.E., W.L. White, J.F. Kelly, R.L. Stout, J.S. Tonigan. "The 10-year course of Alcoholics Anonymous participation and long-term outcomes: a follow-up study of outpatient subjects in Project MATCH." *Substance Abuse: Official Publication of the Association for Medical Education and Research in Substance Abuse* 34, no. 1 (2013):51–59.

199. White, W. *Slaying the Dragon, The History of Addiction Treatment and Recovery in America.* Bloomington, IL: The Chestnut Health Systems, 1998.

200. Prologo, J.D. "Percutaneous CT-Guided Cryovagotomy." *Techniques in Vascular and Interventional Radiology* 23, no. 1 (2020):100660.

201. Martin, M.B., B.T. Hoxworth, D.H. Newman, E.M. Wilson, L. Kinsinger, C. Connor. "S043 mythbuster: truncal vagotomy and gastric drainage procedures." *Surgical Endoscopy* 35, no. 7 (2021):3850–3854.

202. Kral, J.G., W. Paez, B.M. Wolfe. "Vagal nerve function in obesity: therapeutic implications." *World Journal of Surgery* 33, no. 10 (2009):1995–2006.

203. Camilleri, M., J. Toouli, M.F. Herrera, et al. "Intra-abdominal vagal blocking (VBLOC therapy): clinical results with a new implantable medical device." *Surgery* 143, no. 6 (2008):723–731.

204. Nedelec, M, A. McCall, C. Carling, F. Legall, S. Berthoin, G. Dupont. "Recovery in soccer: part II-recovery strategies." *Sports Medicine* 43, no. 1 (2013):9–22.

205. Irwin, M.R., C. Carrillo, R. Olmstead. "Sleep loss activates cellular markers of inflammation: sex differences." *Brain, Behavior, and Immunity* 24, no. 1 (2010):54–57.

206. Vgontzas, A.N., S.Pejovic, E. Zoumakis, et al. "Daytime napping after a night of sleep loss decreases sleepiness, improves performance, and causes beneficial changes in cortisol and interleukin-6 secretion." *American Journal of Physiology Endocrinology and Metabolism* 292, no. 1 (2007):E253–261.

207. Chaves, V.E., F.M. Junior, G.L. Bertolini "The metabolic effects of growth hormone in adipose tissue." *Endocrine* 44, no. 2 (2013):293–302.

208. Golbidi, S., I. Laher. "Exercise induced adipokine changes and the metabolic syndrome." *Journal of Diabetes Research* 2014 (2014):726861.

209. Yang, J. "Enhanced skeletal muscle for effective glucose homeostasis." *Progress in Molecular Biology and Translational Science* 121 (2014):133–163.

210. Kraemer, W.J., B.A. Aguilera, M. Terada, et al. "Responses of IGF-I to endogenous increases in growth hormone after heavy-resistance exercise." *Journal of Applied Physiology* 79, no. 4 (1995):1310–1315.

211. Nishida, Y., T. Matsubara, T. Tobina, et al. "Effect of low-intensity aerobic exercise on insulin-like growth factor-I and insulin-like growth factor-binding proteins in healthy men." *International Journal of Endocrinology* 2010 (2010).

212. Mullington, J.M., M. Haack, M. Toth, J.M. Serrador, H.K. Meier-Ewert. "Cardiovascular, inflammatory, and metabolic consequences of sleep deprivation." *Progress in Cardiovascular Diseases* 51, no. 4 (2009):294–302.

213. Basta, M., G.P. Chrousos, A. Vela-Bueno, A.N. Vgontzas. "Chronic Insomnia and Stress System." *Sleep Medicine Clinics* 2, no. 2 (2007):279–291.

214. St-Onge, M.P. "The role of sleep duration in the regulation of energy balance: effects on energy intakes and expenditure." *Journal of Clinical Sleep Medicine: Official Publication of the American Academy of Sleep Medicine* 9, no. 1 (2013):73–80.

215. Hursel, R., F. Rutters, H.K. Gonnissen, E.A. Martens, M.S. Westerterp-Plantenga. "Effects of sleep fragmentation in healthy men on energy expenditure, substrate oxidation, physical activity, and exhaustion measured over 48 h in a respiratory chamber." *The American Journal of Clinical Nutrition* 94, no. 3 (2011):804–808.

216. Gonnissen, H.K., T. Hulshof, M.S. Westerterp-Plantenga. "Chronobiology, endocrinology, and energy- and food-reward homeostasis." *Obesity Reviews: an Official Journal of the International Association for the Study of Obesity* 14, no. 5 (2013):405–416.